Dealing with Death and Dying

Editors

DAVID BUXTON
NATALIE JACOBOWSKI

CHILD AND ADOLESCENT PSYCHIATRIC CLINICS OF NORTH AMERICA

www.childpsych.theclinics.com

Consulting Editor
TODD E. PETERS

October 2018 • Volume 27 • Number 4

ELSEVIER

1600 John F. Kennedy Boulevard • Suite 1800 • Philadelphia, Pennsylvania, 19103-2899

http://www.theclinics.com

CHILD AND ADOLESCENT PSYCHIATRIC CLINICS OF NORTH AMERICA Volume 27, Number 4
October 2018 ISSN 1056–4993, ISBN-13: 978-0-323-63983-5

Editor: Lauren Boyle
Developmental Editor: Kristen Helm

Child and Adolescent Psychiatric Clinics of North America (ISSN 1056-4993) is published quarterly by Elsevier Inc., 360 Park Avenue South, New York, NY 10010-1710. Months of issue are January, April, July, and October. Business and Editorial Offices: 1600 John F. Kennedy Boulevard, Suite 1800, Philadelphia, PA 19103-2899. Periodicals postage paid at New York, NY and additional mailing offices. Subscription prices are $322.00 per year (US individuals), $594.00 per year (US institutions), $100.00 per year (US students), $382.00 per year (Canadian individuals), $723.00 per year (Canadian institutions), $200.00 per year (Canadian students), $439.00 per year (international individuals), $723.00 per year (international institutions), and $200.00 per year (international students). International air speed delivery is included in all *Clinics* subscription prices. All prices are subject to change without notice. **POSTMASTER:** Send address changes to *Child and Adolescent Psychiatric Clinics of North America*, Elsevier Health Sciences Division, Subscription Customer Service, 3251 Riverport Lane, Maryland Heights, MO 63043. **Customer Service: 1-800-654-2452 (U.S. and Canada); 314-447-8871 (outside U.S. and Canada). Fax: 314-447-8029. E-mail:** JournalsCustomer Service-usa@elsevier.com **(for print support) or** journalsonlinesupport-usa@elsevier.com **(for online support).**

Reprints. For copies of 100 or more of articles in this publication, please contact the Commercial Reprints Department, Elsevier Inc., 360 Park Avenue South, New York, New York 10010-1710 Tel.: 212-633-3874; Fax: 212-633-3820, E-mail: reprints@elsevier.com.

Child and Adolescent Psychiatric Clinics of North America is covered in *MEDLINE/PubMed (Index Medicus), ISI, SSCI, Research Alert, Social Search, Current Contents,* and *EMBASE/Excerpta Medica.*

Contributors

CONSULTING EDITOR

TODD E. PETERS, MD, FAPA
Assistant Chief Medical Informatics Officer/Customer Relationship Manager, Associate
Chief of Staff, Department of Psychiatry and Behavioral Sciences, Vanderbilt University
Medical Center, Medical Director for Inpatient Services, Vanderbilt Psychiatric Hospital,
Assistant Professor of Psychiatry and Behavioral Sciences, Vanderbilt University,
Nashville, Tennessee

EDITORS

DAVID BUXTON, MD
Child and Adult Psychiatrist and Palliative Care Physician, CEO, Center for Palliative
Psychiatry, Medical Director, CJW Medical Center Palliative Care, Richmond, Virginia

NATALIE JACOBOWSKI, MD
Psychiatric Consultation Liaison Service, Department of Child Psychiatry and Behavioral
Health Advanced Illness Management (AIM) Team/Palliative Care, Nationwide Children's
Hospital, Columbus, Ohio

AUTHORS

CHERYL S. AL-MATEEN, MD
Professor, Department of Psychiatry, Division of Child and Adolescent Psychiatry, Virginia
Treatment Center for Children, Virginia Commonwealth University School of Medicine,
Richmond, Virginia

EMILY J. ARON, MD
Assistant Professor, Department of Psychiatry, MedStar Georgetown University Hospital,
Washington, DC

SILVANA BARONE, MD
Stavros Niarchos Foundation Fellow in Pediatric Palliative Care, Division of General
Pediatrics and Adolescent Medicine, The Johns Hopkins Hospital, The Johns Hopkins
University, Hecht-Levi Postdoctoral Fellow, Johns Hopkins Berman Institute of Bioethics,
Baltimore, Maryland

JEFF Q. BOSTIC, MD, EdD
Professor, Department of Psychiatry, MedStar Georgetown University Hospital,
Washington, DC

DAVID BUXTON, MD
Child and Adult Psychiatrist and Palliative Care Physician, CEO, Center for Palliative
Psychiatry, Medical Director, CJW Medical Center Palliative Care, Richmond, Virginia

VALENTINA CIMOLAI, MD
Assistant Professor, Department of Psychiatry, Division of Child and Adolescent Psychiatry, Virginia Treatment Center for Children, Virginia Commonwealth University School of Medicine, Richmond, Virginia

SANDRA CLANCY, PhD
Program Manager, Palliative Care Service, Coordinated Care Clinic, MassGeneral Hospital for Children, Boston, Massachusetts

JULIE GOLDSTEIN GRUMET, PhD
Director of Health and Behavioral Health Initiatives, Suicide Prevention Resource Center, Education Development Center, Inc, Washington, DC

LISA HUMPHREY, MD, FAAP, FAAHPM
Director, Hospice and Palliative Medicine, Nationwide Children's Hospital, Assistant Professor, The Ohio State University College of Medicine, Columbus, Ohio

JANIE ITO, M.Div, BCC
Lead Chaplain, Spiritual Care and Clinical Pastoral Education, Children's Hospital Los Angeles, Los Angeles, California

SANSEA JACOBSON, MD
Assistant Professor, Department of Psychiatry, Western Psychiatric Institute and Clinic, UPMC, Pittsburgh, Pennsylvania

DANIELLE JONAS, MSW, LCSW
Palliative Care Support and Bereavement Counselor, Division of Comfort and Palliative Care, Children's Hospital Los Angeles, Los Angeles, California

KATHRYN JONES, MD, PhD
Assistant Professor, Department of Psychiatry, Division of Child and Adolescent Psychiatry, Virginia Treatment Center for Children, Virginia Commonwealth University School of Medicine, Richmond, Virginia

MARSHA JOSELOW, MA, MSW, LICSW
Palliative Care Social Worker, Pediatric Advanced Care Team, Boston Children's Hospital, Dana-Farber Cancer Institute, Boston, Massachusetts

JULIE LINKER, PhD
Assistant Professor, Department of Psychiatry, Division of Child and Adolescent Psychiatry, Virginia Treatment Center for Children, Virginia Commonwealth University School of Medicine, Richmond, Virginia

BETHANY LOCKWOOD, MD, FAAP
Assistant Professor – Clinical, Division of Palliative Medicine, The Ohio State University College of Medicine, Columbus, Ohio

BLYTH LORD, EdM
Executive Director, Courageous Parents Network, Newton, Massachusetts

MARGARET ROSE MAHONEY, BA
Research Assistant, Office of the Clinical Director, National Institute of Mental Health, Bethesda, Maryland

CYNTHIA W. MOORE, PhD
Psychologist, Department of Psychiatry, Massachusetts General Hospital, Assistant Professor of Psychology, Harvard Medical School, Boston, Massachusetts

SUE E. MORRIS, PsyD
Department of Psychosocial Oncology and Palliative Care, Dana-Farber Cancer Institute, Boston Children's Hospital and Brigham and Women's Hospital, Harvard Medical School, Boston, Massachusetts

ANNA C. MURIEL, MD, MPH
Dana-Farber Cancer Institute, Boston Children's Hospital, Harvard Medical School, Boston, Massachusetts

DOROTHY O'KEEFE, MD
Associate Professor, Department of Psychiatry, Division of Child and Adolescent Psychiatry, Virginia Treatment Center for Children, Virginia Commonwealth University School of Medicine, Richmond, Virginia

MARYLAND PAO, MD
Clinical Director and Deputy Scientific Director, National Institute of Mental Health, Bethesda, Maryland

RACHEL RUSCH, MSW, MA
Palliative Care Support and Bereavement Counselor, Division of Comfort and Palliative Care, Children's Hospital Los Angeles, Los Angeles, California

CAITLIN SCANLON, MSW
Palliative Care Social Worker, Integrated Care Management, Palliative Care Team, Riley Hospital for Children, Indiana University Health, Indianapolis, Indiana

SARAH E. SHEA, PhD
Psychologist, Department of Psychiatry, Massachusetts General Hospital, Instructor in Psychology, Harvard Medical School, Boston, Massachusetts

BARBARA M. SOURKES, PhD
Professor of Pediatrics (and by courtesy Psychiatry and Behavioral Sciences), Stanford University School of Medicine, Kriewall-Haehl Director, Pediatric Palliative Care Program, Lucile Packard Children's Hospital Stanford, Palo Alto, California

SARAH TARQUINI, PhD
Dana-Farber Cancer Institute, Boston Children's Hospital, Harvard Medical School, Boston, Massachusetts

YORAM UNGURU, MD, MS, MA
Division of Pediatric Hematology/Oncology, The Herman and Walter Samuelson Children's Hospital at Sinai, Johns Hopkins Berman Institute of Bioethics, Baltimore, Maryland

TAYLOR R. VEST, MSW
Palliative Care MSW Intern, Virginia Commonwealth University, Richmond, Virginia

Contents

Preface: Dealing with Death and Dying   xi

David Buxton and Natalie Jacobowski

Making Meaning After the Death of a Child   xv

Sandra Clancy and Blyth Lord

> Two bereaved mothers recount how they made meaning after the deaths of their children, recounting how opportunities to tell their stories in medical settings enabled them to construct narratives that promoted resilience and a sense of control. Pediatric palliative care can be conceived as opening space for patients and guardians to tell their stories outside of the specifics of illness, so medical teams can work to accommodate families' values and goals, thereby initiating the process of meaning making. Viewing videos of parent stories enables medical trainees to enhance their communications skills, empathy, and compassion.

"Will You Remember Me?": Talking with Adolescents About Death and Dying   511

Maryland Pao and Margaret Rose Mahoney

> This article describes the preparation, rationale, and benefits of talking with adolescents who have life-threatening or life-limiting illness about advance care planning (ACP) and end-of-life concerns in a developmentally sensitive manner. The first step is to ensure that a health care provider is ready to work with adolescents in ACP discussions by taking a self-inventory, learning communication skills, and understanding individual barriers. The authors then outline how to assess patient and family readiness, including developmental, cultural, personal, and psychosocial considerations. Evidence-based techniques for respectfully and productively engaging adolescents in ACP conversations are discussed.

Supporting Children and Families at a Child's End of Life: Pediatric Palliative Care Pearls of Anticipatory Guidance for Families   527

Bethany Lockwood and Lisa Humphrey

> Mental health professionals can play a key role in helping pediatric patients and their families prepare for and endure the death of a child. Impactful interventions include assisting a family's transition toward acceptance of a child's pending death, using prognostication as a tool in emotional preparedness, and education on expectant symptoms to optimize management and sense of caregiver efficacy.

Ethical Issues Around Pediatric Death: Navigating Consent, Assent, and Disagreement Regarding Life-Sustaining Medical Treatment   539

Silvana Barone and Yoram Unguru

> Decisions regarding whether or not to pursue experimental therapies or life-sustaining medical treatment of children with life-limiting illness can be a

significant source of distress and conflict for both families and health care providers. This article reviews the concepts of parental permission (consent), assent, and emerging capacity and how they relate to decision-making for minors with serious illness. Decision-making capacity for adolescents is discussed generally and in the context of emotionally charged situations pertaining to the end of life. Strategies for minimizing conflict in situations of disagreement between children and families are provided.

Children's Artwork: Its Value in Psychotherapy in Pediatric Palliative Care   551

Barbara M. Sourkes

Pediatric palliative care is a comprehensive treatment approach (physical, psychological, social, spiritual) for children living with life-threatening conditions. These patients and siblings, as well as children of ill parents, face extraordinary psychological challenges. Structured art techniques incorporated into psychotherapy can be powerful for children dealing with life-and-death realities. This article provides the rationale, instructions, and examples for 3 techniques that the author has adapted for children facing illness and bereavement. Although these art techniques are simple to administer, they frequently evoke complex and powerful responses and thus are intended for use by or in consultation with mental health professionals.

Parenting with a Life-Limiting Illness   567

Sarah E. Shea and Cynthia W. Moore

Parents with life-threatening illness face unique challenges in their dual roles as patients and parents. They are at risk for depression, parenting stress, and impaired family functioning, and their children are at risk for adjustment difficulties. In addition to treatment of depression and other mental health issues, patients may also benefit from evidence-informed guidance addressing the challenges of parenting while ill. Consultations should be tailored to each family, with consideration of children's developmental stage and temperament. Clinical recommendations for communication about a parent's anticipated death, helping children spend meaningful time with an ill parent, and legacy leaving are provided.

Bereavement After a Child's Death   579

Danielle Jonas, Caitlin Scanlon, Rachel Rusch, Janie Ito, and Marsha Joselow

The death of a child is a heart-wrenching experience that can have a significant impact on parents, siblings, and families while also often having ripple effects throughout the child's community. Pediatric loss has an impact on family structure and dynamics, individual identity formation, and conceptualization as well as professional practice. This article explores bereavement after a child's death through the lens of the family, the parent, the sibling, the forgotten grievers, and the provider.

The "Liaison" in Consultation-Liaison Psychiatry: Helping Medical Staff Cope with Pediatric Death   591

Anna C. Muriel, Sarah Tarquini, and Sue E. Morris

Pediatric consultation-liaison clinicians are well positioned to provide support, guidance, and systemic recommendations about how to help medical clinicians cope with the stresses of working with dying children. Interventions to support sustainability in this work need to occur at the institutional and team-based levels as well as in individual practice. Shared clinical work around challenging cases provides opportunities to engage with medical clinicians about their difficult experiences and provide reflection and support. Psychiatry services may also be in a role of advocating for institutionally based interventions that can help their medical colleagues.

Social Media Consequences of Pediatric Death   599

David Buxton and Taylor R. Vest

Social media is an important access point for engagement of children and adolescents. For individuals with a life-limiting illness or serving as the caregiver for an ill child, social media can be a helpful outlet for support and information gathering. It has democratized the process of being remembered through providing an ongoing account of thoughts, pictures, and videos that theoretically live on forever via a digital legacy. Providers should be familiar with how this new generation uses social media during their illness, after death, and in the bereavement process.

Assisting the School in Responding to a Suicide Death: What Every Psychiatrist Should Know   607

Emily J. Aron, Jeff Q. Bostic, Julie Goldstein Grumet, and Sansea Jacobson

When a child or adolescent dies by suicide, many individuals are affected, most of whom are attending school. Child and adolescent psychiatrists can be called on during the wake of such tragic events to help schools navigate the difficult tasks following a student suicide. Being familiar with suicide postvention guidelines is crucial for anyone involved in managing the events following a student suicide. By understanding the tenets of suicide postvention and resources that are available to schools and clinicians, the tragedy of suicide can also be an opportunity to improve school mental health and suicide prevention.

Clinician Response to a Child Who Completes Suicide   621

Cheryl S. Al-Mateen, Kathryn Jones, Julie Linker, Dorothy O'Keefe, and Valentina Cimolai

Although suicide is a leading cause of death for children and adolescents, there is a dearth of literature on clinician responses to suicides in that age group. However, most psychiatrists experience the death of a patient by suicide, with resulting grief reactions, including shock, isolation, rumination, self-doubt, and impact on clinical decision making. The impact is more pronounced in trainee clinicians. Postvention is the clinical, administrative, legal, and emotional processes following a suicide. These processes are discussed in detail, with recommendations for policies and training that assist clinicians with this tragic, but common, professional crisis.

CHILD AND ADOLESCENT PSYCHIATRIC CLINICS

FORTHCOMING ISSUES

January 2019
Neuromodulation in Child and Adolescent Psychiatry
Jonathan Essary Becker,
Christopher Todd Maley,
Elizabeth Shultz, and Todd E. Peters,
Editors

April 2019
The Science of Well-Being: Integration into Clinical Child Psychiatry
Jeffrey Bostic, David Rettew, and Matthew Biel, *Editors*

July 2019
Depression in Special Populations
Karen Dineen Wagner and
Warren Y.K. Ng, *Editors*

RECENT ISSUES

July 2018
Emergency Child and Adolescent Psychiatry
Vera Feuer, *Editor*

April 2018
Youth Internet Habits and Mental Health
Kristopher Kaliebe and Paul Weigle,
Editors

January 2018
Co-occurring Medical Illnesses in Child and Adolescent Psychiatry: Updates and Treatment Considerations
Matthew D. Willis, *Editor*

ISSUE OF RELATED INTEREST

Psychiatric Clinics of North America, June 2017 (Vol. 40, No. 2)
Women's Mental Health
Susan G. Kornstein and Anita H. Clayton, *Editors*
Available at: http://www.psych.theclinics.com/

AACAP Members: Please go to www.jaacap.org for information on access to the Child and Adolescent Psychiatric Clinics. *Resident* Members of AACAP: Special access information is available at www.childpsych.theclinics.com.

THE CLINICS ARE AVAILABLE ONLINE!
Access your subscription at:
www.theclinics.com

Preface

Dealing with Death and Dying

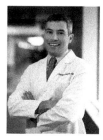 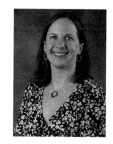

David Buxton, MD   Natalie Jacobowski, MD
Editors

Over the past year, the topic of dying and death has been at the forefront of American news. Events such as the Black Lives Matter movement, the deadliest shooting massacre in US history in Las Vegas, and another school shooting in Florida have speared headlines. It has forced parents, schools, and politicians to speak up about safety, mental health, and death. Children and adolescents have not been sheltered from this topic but, at times, they have been at the center of it with a subsequent increase in many of them having to wrestle with their personal friends' and family's mortality. This phenomenon has led to more questions in the psychological and psychiatric fields on when and how to discuss death with a younger population.

While these sources of death are prominent in the media, the majority of the deaths of the 55,000 children who die each year in America take place in the hospital setting.[1] Often the cause of death includes a mixture of congenital abnormalities, unintentional injuries, malignant neoplasms, suicide, and homicide.[2] The field of palliative care attempts to bridge a gap of integrated psychological and physical care for patients, not only at the end of life but also for patients who have life-limiting illnesses as they still receive more curative-focused treatment. Their treatment includes symptom management, care for physical, emotional, and spiritual suffering, facilitating goals of care conversation, and bereavement support. A majority of the providers entering this specialty are from the field of pediatrics with limited mental health training. It is clear that the psychological effects of complex illnesses and/or acute tragic deaths can be enormous for patients and families as well as for medical providers. When pediatric palliative care is not available, it may be the child psychiatrist who is called upon to support the family or medical teams in the setting of a child's terminal illness. Even when palliative care is available, child and adolescent psychiatrists offer a

Child Adolesc Psychiatric Clin N Am 27 (2018) xi–xiii
https://doi.org/10.1016/j.chc.2018.07.010
1056-4993/18/© 2018 Published by Elsevier Inc.

childpsych.theclinics.com

perspective and skillset that can both benefit families. They can provide valuable education and consultation to pediatric palliative care colleagues who frequently navigate the waters of families' and medical teams' psychological and emotional distress.

Children and adolescents can be also affected by the death of their siblings and parents. The loss of a loved one can be traumatic, leading to developmental stunting and changes in an individual's life trajectory. In fact, there is a famous example of this concept in the possible shaping of one of psychiatry's forefathers, Sigmund Freud. In one of his less known publications, he discussed the impact of the death of his six-month-old brother, Julius, when Freud was two years old. The loss resonated throughout his childhood as, at the time, his mother was already grieving from the death of her own younger brother who had died of tuberculosis one month before she gave birth to baby Julius. Her grief and depression were further augmented by this double loss, which left her even more emotionally unavailable to Sigmund. He wrote about the impact of this in his self-analysis: "I greeted my one year-younger brother, who died after a few months, with adverse wishes and genuine childhood jealousy…his death left the germ of self reproaches in me."[3] The losses of these family members and the deleterious psychological impact they both directly and indirectly had on him may have catalyzed his quest to understand the human psyche.

The idea for this issue of *Child and Adolescent Psychiatric Clinics of North America* stemmed from a lack of concise psychological resources related to death and dying in pediatrics. The framework was designed to approach the topic from multiple angles to provide a broad spectrum on how dying and death can affect individuals, providers, families, and systems. We are honored to have specialists from across the country discuss these difficult topics and to have a special editorial by parents who have lost a child, sharing their unique perspectives on death and dying in pediatrics. The multidisciplinary expertise provided will highlight clinical practices and possible strategies to help transverse a difficult time in all human lives. Our hope is that readers gain greater understanding and appreciation of how child and adolescent psychiatry can play a major role in easing suffering for individuals and systems during death and dying.

David Buxton, MD
Center for Palliative Psychiatry
2000 Bremo Road
Suite 100
Richmond, VA 23226, USA

Natalie Jacobowski, MD
Psychiatric Consultation Liaison Service
Department of Child Psychiatry and
Behavioral Health Advanced Illness Management Team/
Palliative Care
Nationwide Children's Hospital
190 South High Street #295
Columbus, OH 43215, USA

E-mail addresses:
dbuxton@palliativepsychiatry.com (D. Buxton)
natalie.jacobowski@nationwidechildrens.org (N. Jacobowski)

REFERENCES

1. Keele L, Keenan HT, Sheetz J, et al. Differences in characteristics of dying children who receive and do not receive palliative care. Pediatrics 2013;132:72–8.
2. Murphy SL, Xu J, Kochanek KD, et al. Deaths: final data for 2015. National vital statistics reports. Vol. 66. No. 6. November 27, 2017. Available at: https://www.cdc.gov/nchs/data/nvsr/nvsr66/nvsr66_06.pdf. Accessed July 31, 2018.
3. Breger L. Freud: darkness in the midst of vision. New York: John Wiley & Sons; 2000. p. 10–3.

Making Meaning After the Death of a Child

Sandra Clancy, PhD[a],*, Blyth Lord, EdM[b]

KEYWORDS

- Pediatric palliative care • Bereavement • Patient experience • Medical storytelling
- Medical education • Patient voice

KEY POINTS

- Two bereaved mothers articulate how they made meaning after the deaths of their children.
- Opportunities to share their experiences in medical settings helped them construct narratives of resilience and a sense of control.
- Pediatric palliative care can be conceived of as a way to provide space for patients and parents to tell their stories outside of the specifics of illness, thereby initiating the process of meaning making.
- Viewing video interviews of parents of children with serious illnesses allows medical trainees to understand the parent perspective and hear their stories, enhancing trainees' communications skills, empathy and compassion.

INTRODUCTION

This article is a story of stories. It begins as 2 individual stories, as told by Blyth and Sandy, about caring for children with rare and life-limiting illnesses. These paths then join together to become a third story that, as it unfolds, gathers up the stories of many other families. All of the families and their stories are different in the ways that families differ, but the essential subjects and themes are similar and formidable: the life and death of a beloved child from serious illness, the quiet thirst for meaning that follows, and the gradual construction of that meaning over time.

Making meaning is a universal human endeavor, but for a parent whose child has died, the enterprise takes on urgency and focus. Sandy and Blyth were finding meaning in nurturing their children and looking forward to the normal milestones all parents anticipate. With the radical disruption of losing their young children, every aspect of

Disclosure Statement: No disclosures.
[a] Palliative Care Service, Coordinated Care Clinic, MassGeneral Hospital for Children, 175 Cambridge Street, Boston, MA 02114, USA; [b] Courageous Parents Network, 21 Rochester Road, Newton, MA 02458, USA
* Corresponding author.
E-mail address: sclancy2@mgh.harvard.edu

their lives changed and the excruciating questions arose: Is there a meaning to my life now or is there different meaning to my life, now that my child has died? And if so, what is it?

For both women, the journey toward reconstructing meaning began with the simple impulse to tell the story of what happened, sharing with medical providers and other parents who had experienced the death of a child. Their efforts have resulted in a profound friendship borne of shared experience, collaboration around advocacy for pediatric palliative care, and innovative work in medical education. The culmination of both their journeys is the belief that it is through story that all parents can find their meaning, along with growth, resilience, self-compassion, and a sense of control.

BLYTH LORD'S STORY

"The world was broken and the three of us—mother, father, son—were falling into its mouth." This line from Emily Rapp's grief memoir *The Still Point of the Turning World*,[1] written in the first year after she learns that her infant son has Tay-Sachs and will die sometime in the next few years, resonates so completely with me because it was exactly how I felt when I learned that my second daughter, Cameron, had Tay-Sachs. Except in our case the line would read, The 7 of us were falling into its mouth, that is, 2 fathers, 2 mothers, the 2 children, and 1 sibling.

In 1999 my 18-month-old nephew Hayden was diagnosed with infantile Tay-Sachs. One month later, my 6-month-old daughter Cameron was diagnosed with the same disease. Tay-Sachs is a rare and incurable genetic illness that always ends in early childhood death. Both parents must be carriers of the gene. Hayden and Cameron's fathers are identical twins, unknowing carriers who both married unknowing carriers—women who were best friends in college. The twins' genetic mutation had never been seen before, and the likelihood of these two brothers marrying carriers and having affected children was 1 in 80,000,000. What happened in our family was a statistical near impossibility.

But, in its way, it made everything that followed possible.

My husband Charlie and I and our brother and sister-in-law, Tim and Alison, were traveling together on the road toward our respective children's deaths. We were also traveling the distance together to figure out how to cope. Our children would be beloved. We would give them the best lives possible and then prepare to give them the best deaths possible. And we would pray that we survived.

We did more than survive. Despite the profound sadness of watching our beautiful daughter lose all cognitive and physical abilities, Charlie and I were able to live fully into Cameron's short life and to help Cameron's big sister Taylor, 4 years old, understand it as best she could. Despite the fear we had of losing Cameron, we became prepared to accept, face, and allow her pending death. Shortly after Cameron's diagnosis, Charlie bravely declared that Cameron's life would have a full arc, with a beginning and a middle and an end. We would do the best we could to live into that arc and to make the ending a good one.

I give much credit to the gifted psychologist, serving as a grief counselor with whom we worked during Cameron's life, for our ability to construct and own this vision of an arc to the point where it felt like destiny. She shepherded us as we processed our anticipatory grief following the diagnosis, and she helped us begin to put the pieces together so that Cameron's death was not a tragedy that was happening to our family. Rather, she helped us look at the experience in all of its facets, matching the sadness with the joy and the loss with the personal growth that we could feel happening even in her office. If I had to tell you where the tone was set for our story, I would say it was set there, with me and Charlie and the counselor in her office a few months after the diagnosis. And it grew from there.

Charlie was with Tim and Alison for the last few days of Hayden's life and was able to tell me that Hayden was comfortable, that the death was peaceful, that Tim and Alison were OK, and that we were going to be OK when our time came. He had been there and I believed him, which made such a difference. And despite the whoosh that poured from our life and our home when we watched Cameron die 5 months later, we were able to process our grief and slowly emerge from the grief cave intact and alert.

I use this word *alert* because I was on the lookout. Given the statistical improbability of what had happened and the magnitude of these two beautiful babies dying so young from such a rare disease, I was certain that something more was supposed to grow of this experience and that I must pay attention so that I recognized it when I saw it. Clichéd as this sounds, I have come to think of the process of *meaning making* and its sister *transformational growth* like that of a seed that puts roots down and then, with time and space, shoots up and up until it presents itself as the tree it has become. (And honestly, what is more reassuring than the natural world and nature as a model for life, for living?) I knew what the seed was. Now I was looking for the growth.

The immediate sign of life was that we, Hayden and Cameron's parents and grandparents, started a small family foundation the year after they died. For 17 years now, the foundation has raised funds from family and friends, and it gives annual grants to support pediatric palliative care programs and research and to fund medical research for a treatment of Tay-Sachs.

Charlie and I then began telling our story. We had first told our story when our unusual situation was featured in PBS's NOVA 2001 2-hour special on the Human Genome Project, for which the 4 parents were interviewed and the children videotaped. The program aired in the period between Hayden's death and Cameron's, and I remember feeling like we were somehow in no-man's-land, exposed and waiting publicly for what everyone now knew was coming.

A year after Cameron's death, we began to tell the story in a new way, to a new audience: talking to medical students and residents about how our daughter's primary care pediatrician worked with us during Cameron's lifetime. We described how this doctor delivered the diagnosis, gave anticipatory guidance, helped us identify our care goals and values, and then accompanied us through Cameron's transition to end of life and, most enduringly, how his care, which was almost entirely palliative care, made such a difference. After telling the story upwards of 6 times, I began to worry that something so sacred was becoming rote and worn, and so we partnered with the American Academy of Pediatrics to produce it as a minidocumentary and training video called *Cameron's Arc.* The video is about the role a primary care pediatrician can play in ensuring that the arc is a good one, and it is distributed to pediatric residency programs around the country.

In talking to the medical students and producing *Cameron's Arc*, I experienced firsthand the therapeutic nature of storytelling in the face of grief and child loss. I felt myself turning toward this in my own growth. I also found myself wanting to help other parents tell their story. Partnering with National Tay-Sachs and Allied Disease association (NTSAD) in a volunteer capacity (disclosure: I have recently been elected President of the NTSAD Board of Directors), I produced the video *Parenting a Child with Life-Threatening Illness* for distribution to newly diagnosed families. In this video, 5 couples share their experiences from coping with the diagnosis, tending the marriage, caring for the siblings, managing symptoms, developing a philosophy of care, and transitioning to end of life with their child. I loved giving a voice to these families and knowing that they were helping other parents who were following.

In listening to these parents, I also learned the power of being an audience for another person's story of loss and grief and, in so doing, helping them incorporate the loss into their family narrative. In an interview about 'listening generously' in the context of chronic illness and the practice of medicine, Rachel Naomi Remen stresses, "The story is the container for meaning."[2] Within a few years, I recognized storytelling as the direction I wanted to go in to help make meaning of Cameron and Hayden's lives and deliver on what, with increasing urgency, I was now feeling as my obligation to *do something more*.

This pulsing certainty that I was obligated to *do something more* was accompanied by a pressing fear that I was going to never figure it out and that I was going to fail: fail my daughter, my nephew, their magic, myself, and the fellow parents who were currently going through it. My full-time job in television production at WGBH/PBS was a wonderful one but it was not *it*. One fateful day, as I traveled back from Florida with our daughter's pediatrician following a weekend presentation we had given on *Cameron's Arc* and pediatric palliative care at a conference, I turned to him and asked, "What am I supposed to do?" He responded, "Play the cards you're holding." On a yellow legal pad, right there on the plane, I listed those cards and diagrammed how they connected to each other: serious illness in children, storytelling, video production, distance learning, Web design, palliative care, grief counseling, bereavement.

In 2013, 6 months after that plane ride and 11 years after Cameron's death, I left my job in television production to develop, launch, and dedicate myself full-time to Courageous Parents Network (CPN). CPN is a nonprofit whose mission it is to empower, guide, and support parents caring for children with life-threatening illness. Our digital resources shine a light on the difficult issues that families face to help them find their way. Through blog posts, audio podcasts, and nearly 500 short videos (80% parent voices, 20% provider voices), CPN provides guidance from parents and professionals on such topics as understanding anticipatory grief, genetic counseling, palliative care, and talking with children about death. It gives parents insights and knowledge from other parents who have gone before on topics that include adapting to the diagnosis, tending to the marriage, coping with fear of regrets, caring for the other children, making difficult decisions about medical interventions, and finding meaning and identity after the child dies.

Hayden died in December 2000 and Cameron died in May 2001. Seventeen years later, I am in the flow of what their lives and deaths germinated. CPN is the mature phase of my own growth and the manifestation of how I have made meaning and incorporated it into my life. Importantly, it is not about my daughter or family. That was the seed from which it grew, but it is now grafted onto those of all the other families that have walked (or are walking) this path.

Parents caring for children with life-threatening illnesses and bereaved parents are a special community—not as rare as we would like, of course, but rare enough that we tend to find each other. And on my path toward Courageous Parents Network, I found Sandy and she found me.

SANDY'S STORY

If you had asked me at the time of my 5-year old son Jack's death whether I could make any meaning of it, I would have been offended by the question. I would have articulated a resounding and very clear NO. I was too stunned by what had happened to be able to piece any coherent narrative together or look beyond the day. But over the years, the impulse to tell the story, both to myself and others, along with my collaborations with Blyth, have opened up the possibility of making meaning. As Blyth so beautifully articulated, meaning making begins with telling the story; I would add retelling, refining, reflecting, listening to others, refining again and again and again until it becomes—and for me, *became*—fully and completely a very individual story.

There are many stories within the story. I will start by making clear that I cannot possibly tell the story of Jack's experience. He became very sick at 5 years of age and died 9 months later. Although we supported and loved him beyond the limits of our abilities, I cannot imagine what he truly thought, felt, and experienced. Likewise, I have heard and appreciated doctors telling Jack's story from a medical point of view. Indeed, I have sometimes repeated the medical story, although not with the precision and knowledge of a doctor.

No, this story is about the journey my husband and I took, while caring for our seriously ill child, in a medical setting. Because of the circumstance of Jack's illness and death, the fact that he got sick so fast and we were consumed into a medical system, medicine is a dominant character in the story that at times controlled us to the point where we did what it required, trying desperately to work within it to save his life. Perhaps it was inevitable that we followed the demands of the medical system given that Jack was undiagnosed for 8 months, that he received care in a major academic medical center that, on diagnosis, developed a laserlike focus on cure until cure was declared impossible just a week before Jack died. The journey my husband and I took was one of survival and not much reflection, leaving us exhausted, numb, traumatized, and feeling like shells of human beings.

Over the years, in the telling of the story, I now see that the seeds of meaning were sown in those hospital experiences with Jack, and it is there where I begin this story.

In January of 2004, Jack was a healthy, active, engaged preschooler. He began to have severe headaches and stomachaches just around the time of his fifth birthday. I brought him to see his primary care physician many times after episodes of extreme pain. Unable to find any cause for the symptoms, the doctor suggested that I make an appointment with a child psychiatrist to investigate whether anxiety was a factor. The psychiatrist encouraged me to continue to pursue a medical workup given his opinion that there was some organic cause for the symptoms.

Finally, Jack's pediatrician observed papilledema, a condition in which increased pressure in and around the brain causes part of the optic nerve to swell and create many of Jack's presenting symptoms. Our physician sent us to an emergency department, where imaging showed a subdural hygroma, an abnormal accumulation of cerebrospinal fluid. A neurosurgeon performed a burr hole procedure, which drained the fluid; we were sent home with the hope that a trauma to the head or a type of meningitis had caused the fluid and that it would not come back. Unfortunately, it returned in a couple of days and the neurosurgeon placed a ventriculoperitoneal shunt.

Over the next 8 months, Jack underwent what one doctor called "a million-dollar workup" overseen by the many subspecialists who joined his team: doctors from neurology, rheumatology, infectious disease, gastroenterology, hematology/oncology, neurosurgery and many others. Our 5 year old had blood draws, biopsies, and imaging, among many other procedures. He experienced innumerable outpatient appointments, many trips to the emergency department for pain and questions of shunt malfunction, in-patient stays for various viruses and infections, and pediatric intensive care unit (PICU) stays after procedures. The distressing experience was made worse by the fact that the care he received at one of the best hospitals in the world was fragmented, most especially in the outpatient setting. Individual providers did everything they could to improve the quality of Jack's life and ultimately to save it, but they operated within a system that did not enable them to do so effectively.

There was no clear medical team leader, and individual providers often focused on one organ system or part of the body. It became apparent that communication among providers was difficult, and my husband and I were left as the repositories of *the whole story*. We were challenged by these systems' defects, the unrelenting nature of Jack's illness that left him in pain, frail, and exhausted, and the fact that we had a steep learning curve in navigating a medical system and culture that required acquiring a new language and skills.

In early August of 2004, Jack was admitted to the hospital for the last time and was eventually diagnosed with Degos disease (also known as Kohlmeier-Degos disease or malignant atrophic papulosis), an extraordinarily rare blood vessel disorder. For the next 2 months, we participated in and observed a valiant effort to find a cure. Although the experience was harrowing, at least we had some sense of order. The Chief of the Pediatric Service became the identified leader of the medical team; in what proved to be crucial to our experience, he made clear to my husband and me that we too were vital and necessary members of that team. Our expertise was knowing our son well, thereby granting us a status that we had previously lacked.

Being recognized as equal participants in Jack's medical care mattered a great deal to us in many ways. It really changed how we interacted with providers and they with us. Moreover, when Jack died, it was not a loss that we experienced alone, because we truly felt part of an extraordinary collaboration. We received an enormous amount of support in the hospital from a wonderful child psychiatrist and her resident who visited us most days. Sometimes one or the other stayed with us in silence as we endured watching a procedure, or they joined team meetings, or we managed 10 minutes of dialogue in between important subspecialist visits. They helped us with how to talk to our younger son and to our elderly parents and supported us to sometimes stand firm and insist on asking physicians questions that they clearly did not want to answer. The overnight nurses listened to our observations, questions, and concerns and gave us honest answers even if they did not accord with the medical team's consensus. There were also the residents who lived in the hospital with us, several of whom we learned had experienced the loss of a parent or sibling. I felt an odd camaraderie with these smart and intense young people who, too, were learning a new system and had so much responsibility and yet were open to the emotional aspects and allowed themselves to care deeply for my family.

I have come to appreciate that the Chief of Pediatrics, by formally recognizing us as part of Jack's medical team and encouraging us to share our experiences of care, opened space for us to tell our and Jack's story and begin the process of making meaning.

My husband and I asked to meet with the chief 2 weeks after Jack died in order to thank him. We also sought to delineate how the fragmentation of care we had experienced, especially when we were home with Jack, turned us into case managers and how this made it hard for us to simply spend time with him and be parents throughout his ordeal.

At our meeting the chief not only fully acknowledged the problems we articulated but also introduced us to a novel model that had been developed to address them. The Medical Home for Children with Special Healthcare Needs was an idea originated by the American Academy of Pediatrics to better coordinate the care of children with complex medical problems. He asked me to join the hospital's efforts by participating on a committee charged with developing a medical home at the hospital. In this way, my husband and I had a concrete way to address the problems we had experienced.

It was on this committee that I began to tell my story to a wider audience, relaying our difficulties, and hearing that the physician members themselves also recognized and wanted to ameliorate them. Here was an opportunity to undertake truly meaningful and important work in which my perspective was needed to make a positive impact.

After a year on the planning committee, I joined the Coordinated Care Clinic's team as program manager and I have stayed in this position for 10 years. It is hard for me to express and even comprehend why I agreed to participate in this effort. It was deeply important to me that the project come to fruition and I wanted to ensure that it got off the ground. This effort was serious work, and I felt prepared to do it given what I had experienced.

To all this, I would add the concepts of *making sure no one else experienced what we had* and *helping other people*. However, these do not capture the whole story because this was not an entirely self-less act. It was about processing, understanding, and ultimately making meaning of the devastation that had taken place. Over the years I have told my story many times. In developing and promoting the Coordinated Care Clinic, I used my family's story as an illustration of what many families experience and of how system changes matter. A few years after beginning my work at the hospital, I joined the Pediatric Palliative Care team as Program Manager. I also chair the hospital's Family Advisory Council, all roles in which I interact with families that are caring for children with life-threatening or life–limiting illness.

Most recently I was invited to speak to a Master's Level Medical Social worker class at a local university, telling the story yet again but with a slightly different focus: how my entire family coped throughout the hospital ordeal and beyond. It was in this retelling that I realized again how valuable it is for medical trainees to hear the parent perspective and better understand the reasons parents say and do certain things that otherwise seem puzzling. In a similar vein, I have become involved in efforts with researchers to understand and find treatments for Degos Disease and will participate in an international conference at the National Institutes of Health, explaining what has motivated me to undertake this work and guiding researchers on how to encourage other patients and parents to collaborate in research efforts.

It is in these retellings that I am able to see how far I and my family have come over the last 14 years. As a family, we no longer simply survive. We live fully, with meaning, to honor our son Jack.

THE STORIES COME TOGETHER

We first met at a small dinner party given by a mutual friend. Blyth does not remember being told that Sandy was also a bereaved mom, but there was a noticeable sadness to Sandy that night. When the hostess followed up that Sandy's son Jack had died several years prior, it all made sense. Of course: Sandy was wearing the face of a grieving parent.

Not too long afterward, we met again but this time under professional circumstances, and this is where everything comes together. By this time, Sandy was in position at the hospital and, as part of that, working with the head of pediatric palliative care to build support for this new service. Palliative care was using the videos Blyth had produced, *Cameron's Arc* and *Parenting a Child with Life-Threatening Illnesses*, as a way to bring parent voices and stories into the hospital's medical education program. Sandy also occasionally invited Blyth to join the series of communications workshops she was helping run, wherein residents role-play delivering bad news to parents. At the same time, Blyth was evolving her vision for CPN and asked Sandy to advise. With generosity and wisdom, Sandy became a founding member of CPN's Professional Advisory Board.

We are now linked professionally. Our respective paths have merged. Blyth works full-time as Executive Director at CPN. Sandy works full-time at the hospital and also serves as chair of CPN's Professional Advisory Board. Together, we are professionally dedicated to helping parents caring for children with life-threatening illness. We are committed to empowering parents while their child is living; we especially advocate for pediatric palliative care as care that fills gaps and offers psychosocial and emotional support stretching out beyond curative treatments to focus on quality of life for the entire family. We are involved in an innovative medical education project using CPN videos to help introduce the parent perspective outside of the clinical setting, allowing trainees to reflect on difficult conversations and process their own emotions around the serious illness of patients. And we are committed to supporting parents and helping them in their process of finding meaning and identity after their child dies.

WHAT WE HAVE LEARNED

Flannery O'Connor is purported to have said: "I write because I don't know what I think until I read what I say." We tell our stories because we do not know how far we have come and what we did for our children until we hear what we say. There is no sense to be made of the death of a child. Instead, what one can hope for is that, with time, a family has the opportunity to put the pieces together into a flow that is palatable enough that they can live with it, live into it, and go on. Of course, everyone has a story. But in the cases of serious illness in children, when death is a possibility or certainty, we see an opportunity and feel an obligation to try to help families begin organizing the pieces in anticipation of their story *ahead of time*. The goal is that after their child has died, as they are reflecting back, parents and other family members are already primed to see the distance they have traveled, the milestones along the way, and the courage and strengths they brought. If we can help families fit the pieces together, they are likely to have a greater sense of control in a larger narrative that was entirely out of their control. This idea is the purview of personal narrative and palliative care, two resources we promote with the families we work with today. *The better the before, the better the after*.

We are social beings and the act of framing one's own difficult experience so as to help others feels life affirming and purposeful. It is also a Trojan horse for the healing that comes with meaning making. CPN has interviewed dozens of parents: some are single mothers, most are a mother and father pair, half are bereaved within the past 24 months, and half are currently caring for their ill child. Most have other, healthy children; a few are parenting more than one very ill child. In each interview, regardless of whether the child is living or deceased, parents convey the meaning they have found in their experience. During the interview, the parents give shape and voice to their child's and family's story, molding and presenting it as one of coping and surviving. In giving these families an audience, CPN is helping to validate their story. Such validation in turn helps the family recreate their identity and sense of agency and helps parents reinvest in a world where it is possible for a child to die. As one mother interviewed said afterward: "It was good to look at the journey from the beginning and from all aspects. It was encouraging to me to encourage other families. It brought the whole journey together... The interview made me put my feelings into words. It made me think about other people. Most of all, as I reflected on the highs and lows of this journey, I realized how strong I was, and I was thankful God was with me through it all."

Storytelling is accessible to everyone. It does not ask the family member to make any grand gestures, like starting a foundation or building a playground in their child's name. Rather, it directs parents to position themselves as people who did the best they could with what they had in the face of extreme difficulty and who survived and can look ahead. Certainly, this is evident in our two examples and there are countless others.[a] Through the storytelling, parents absorb, in a deeper way, all they did to be good parents, which our own experience as well as research indicates is vital to helping parents emotionally survive.[3]

We two bereaved mothers, plus dozens of other parents we have met, are advocates for pediatric palliative care for children living with serious illness because palliative care too helps position both patients and family members as empowered actors in the story. Although the official definition does not mention storytelling, palliative care, in fact, encourages and invites parents and children to tell their story outside the specifics of illness so that medical teams can accommodate a family's values and meaning. As part of this process, providers are intentional about giving parents figurative space to reflect on their role as caregiver and decision-maker, and support them in making those decisions they consider best, because this makes a significant difference in how the family collectively remembers. In a piece for *The New Yorker*[4] on pediatric palliative care ("Lives Less Ordinary", 1/20/14), Dr Jerome Groopman quotes Janet Duncan, a pediatric palliative care nurse, as she acknowledges the proclivity of some parents to experience self-recrimination and regret following the death of their child: "We are often the ones to help these families remember that they went through a very thoughtful, careful process of what would help their child live as well as possible, and they did the very best they could with the information they had."

We are also strong advocates for professional psychological support to help parents process their anticipatory grief, validate and normalize their emotions, and understand their relationship in the context of their child's illness. We both benefited from such support: as noted earlier, Blyth and her husband working closely with a psychologist for nearly 3 years, from diagnosis through the first year of bereavement, and Sandy and her husband working with a psychiatrist and her resident who initially joined the team to work with Jack. As Jack grew sicker and unable to communicate, they helped in a variety of ways during the long hospital stays. They helped Sandy and her husband process their emotions on a daily basis, brainstormed around managing interactions with family and friends, and offered advice about communicating with their other son. They continued to be available for meetings and phone calls after Jack's death. It is not an exaggeration for both Blyth and Sandy to wonder what would have become of their families if these smart and compassionate people had not been involved in their care.

It is worth noting, however, that intelligent, wise, experienced counselors for this difficult terrain are hard to find. It is our hope that more psychologists and psychiatrists gain expertise in this special field of pediatric illness and death and are there to accompany parents on this life-changing journey. It is difficult but noble work that has a lasting impact on how the family remembers and tells the story.

---

[a] A colleague in the United Kingdom, Sacha Langton-Gilks, is the mother of DD who died of cancer at 16 years of age. Her recently published book Follow the Child: Planning and Having the Best End-of Life Care for Your Child (Jessica Kingsley Publishers, London, 2018) is part memoir and part surreal how-to, in which she shares in intense but safe detail the ups and downs of her own journey with DD so as to help parents anticipating their child's end of life. In an interview with The Guardian (digital version, January 20, 2018), she says, "My biggest consolation in grief and my greatest achievement in life is to have fulfilled the wishes of my child—emotional, physical, spiritual—as he approached death during the last three months after his terminal diagnosis. I do not have guilt or questions and I know full well how lucky I am to be able to say that. I have met families who did not have this and they tell me they will never recover and, knowing what DD's good death means to me, I believe them." https://www.theguardian.com/lifeandstyle/2018/jan/21/iwatched-my-son-die-from-cancer-lessons-i-have-learned-sacha-langton-gilks

SUMMARY

In writing this piece, we have both struggled with the limits of language (and our writing prowess) to capture something that is so intimate and painful and organic and powerful. It is hard to write honestly and with complexity about events that are so difficult and to find just the right metaphors. For example, it is unquestionably satisfying to know that improvements one has participated in bringing to fruition make it easier for the next family. As noted, however, this is not pure altruism. Also driving our work is the parallel impulse for understanding and self-knowledge that comes from the desire to address the seismic effect of the death of a child.

We note that this is really a job for a poet. We are not poets. We are parents with formal educations and avocations in other things entirely, redirected to do serious and important work with good people, fellow parents and medical providers, who are pouring themselves into the inspiring act of living in the face of illness and death in children. The enterprise of making meaning in life is one that all human beings undertake at some level, whether intentionally or not. Our experiences have been utterly transformative and they have reshaped our lives. It makes the utmost sense to us that we two bereaved mothers have endeavored, personally and professionally, to make this particular sense from our losses. We wish for other parents the ability to construct their story, their meaning, one that helps them to go on and face each day with hope and resilience.

REFERENCES

1. Rapp E. The still point of the turning world. New York: Penguin Books; 2013. p. 4.
2. Remen RN. Listening generously. On being with Krista Tippet. July 10, 2010. Available at: onbeing.org/programs/rachel-naomi-remen-listening-generously/. Accessed July 19, 2018.
3. Hinds PS, Oakes LL, Hicks J, et al. "Trying to be a good parent" as defined by interviews with parents who made phase I, terminal care, and resuscitation decisions for their children. J Clin Oncol 2009;27:5979–85.
4. Groopman J. Lives less ordinary. New York: The New Yorker; January 20, 2014.

"Will You Remember Me?"
Talking with Adolescents About Death and Dying

Maryland Pao, MD[a],*, Margaret Rose Mahoney, BA[b]

KEYWORDS

- Adolescents • Advance care planning • Decision-making • End-of-life
- Palliative care

KEY POINTS

- Talking with adolescents who have a life-threatening or life-limiting illness is one of the most difficult tasks a health care provider (HCP) can undertake.
- A necessary and important first step in learning how to speak with adolescents about death or dying is assessing one's own readiness as an HCP.
- Adolescents want to be included in medical decision-making through the illness trajectory including making decisions around end-of-life.
- Prognosis is not necessary before initiating advance care planning discussions.

INTRODUCTION

Talking with adolescents who have a life-threatening or life-limiting illness is one of the most difficult tasks a health care provider (HCP) can undertake. In the past, medical providers, parents, and the public have thought that conversations about dying, advance care planning (ACP), and end-of-life discussions should be avoided with medically ill youth.[1] This was due to a desire to protect children and adolescents or due to beliefs that they do not understand death and dying or do not have the capacity to make decisions about their own health. However, modern Western society has come to understand that these difficult conversations are not only often beneficial for patients and families but also are increasingly considered the standard of care. Today, the American Academy of Pediatrics,[2] the Institute of Medicine,[3] and the World Health Organization[4] recommend involving youth in decisions regarding their health

Disclosure Statement: No disclosures.
[a] National Institute of Mental Health, 10 Center Drive MSC 1276, NIH Building 10 CRC 6-5340, Bethesda, MD 20892-1276, USA; [b] Office of the Clinical Director, National Institute of Mental Health, 10 Center Drive MSC 1276, NIH Building 10 CRC 6-5360, Bethesda, MD 20892-1276, USA
* Corresponding author.
E-mail address: paom@mail.nih.gov

Child Adolesc Psychiatric Clin N Am 27 (2018) 511–526
https://doi.org/10.1016/j.chc.2018.05.001
1056-4993/18/Published by Elsevier Inc.

childpsych.theclinics.com

care decisions as they are developmentally and emotionally ready. This article focuses on the following:

1. Adolescents who have a life-limiting condition and their understanding of death,
2. Developmental considerations around health care decisions, and
3. A practical approach to engaging adolescents in conversations around ACP, including addressing barriers to communication, especially at the end-of-life (**Fig. 1**).[5]

HISTORICAL PERSPECTIVE

As recently as the 1970s, revealing a cancer diagnosis to a child was considered inhumane. Researchers believed that children and adolescents were not aware of their impending deaths and that the stigma of a cancer diagnosis should not be shared

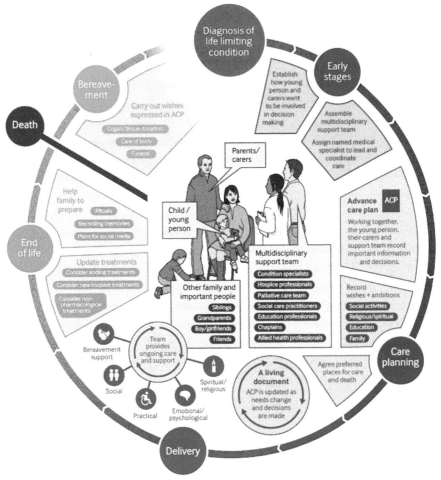

Fig. 1. End-of-life care for children and young people. (*From* Villanueva G, Murphy MS, Vickers D, et al. End of life care for infants, children and young people with life limiting conditions: summary of NICE guidance. BMJ 2016;355:i6385; with permission.)

with them. However, as researchers began talking, drawing, and playing with children in hospitals, they began to notice that even sick young children were aware of their illness and would conceal knowledge of their impending death from their parents at the same time the parents were attempting to suppress any discussion about the child's serious illness in the "maintenance of mutual pretense."[6,7] By the early 2000s, a survey study by Kreicbergs and colleagues[8] on parents who had lost a child to cancer in the 1990s showed that none of the group of parents who had talked with their child about death regretted it, but 27% who did not talk with their child about death regretted not having done so. Parents who had sensed their child was aware of imminent death were more likely to regret not talking than those who had not sensed awareness in their child. Mothers were more likely to regret than fathers, as were parents of older children compared with parents of younger children. Parents who had talked with their children were more likely to have sensed their child was aware of imminent death and were more often religious, older, and had older children. In addition, concurrent with major advances in medical technology and increased survivorship of many chronic childhood illnesses, such as sickle cell disease, cystic fibrosis, cardiac anomalies, and childhood leukemia, a burgeoning movement for palliative care for the dying adolescent began taking place at pediatric hospitals and cancer programs.[9,10]

HEALTH CARE PROVIDER READINESS

An individual's own cultural and emotional experience with death will influence their ability and confidence in talking about dying with other people. Physicians and other HCPs frequently express uncertainty about how to address ACP, or involvement in medical decision-making throughout the course of the illness, primarily due to concerns about taking away hope from patients and their families. Therefore, a necessary and important first step in learning how to speak with adolescents about death or dying is assessing one's own readiness to do so as a HCP.

Take a Self-Inventory

HCPs need to understand their personal feelings about death in order to be effective in providing support to adolescents who are facing their own impending death. HCPs are encouraged to take a self-inventory periodically throughout their medical education and practice to understand their own perception of death and its evolution over time as they mature. Each person's experiences with death will inform the way they interact with others regarding death. This introspection can be done both formally and informally. In *Grief, Dying, and Death: Clinical Interventions for Caregivers* (1984),[11] Therese Rando provides exercises for self-assessment (**Boxes 1** and **2**).

As HCPs are only human, anticipatory grief of inevitable outcomes may lead to avoidance or lack of engagement with dying patients and their families. Self-awareness and self-monitoring of one's own reactions (sometimes referred to as "countertransference") are important areas to examine periodically if one is going to engage consistently in palliative care, especially with youth.[12]

Learn Communication Skills

Parents often do not talk to their child about what is happening in order to protect their child.[13] Despite this, youth, especially adolescents, often know that they are very sick and/or dying. Withholding information about an adolescent's medical status can cause them to suspect that they are more seriously ill, increase sibling suffering, strain the parental relationship, and jeopardize trust. Parents and practitioners alike can help

---

Box 1
Early experiences influencing reactions to loss and death

Our early experiences with loss and death leave us with messages, feelings, fears, and attitudes we will carry throughout life. To prevent our being controlled by our unconscious and conscious reactions to past experiences, it is important to recognize and state explicitly how these experiences have influenced us and our lifestyles.

Think about your earliest death-related experience:

When did it occur? Where was it? Who was involved? What happened?

What were your reactions, positive and negative?

What were you advised to do, and what did you do, to cope with the experience?

What did you learn about death and loss as result of this experience?

Of the things you learned then, what makes you feel fearful or anxious now?

Of the things you learned then, what makes it easier for you to cope with death now?

Think about your own feelings about death and the attitudes you maintain about it currently. Write down these feelings and attitudes.

The feelings and attitudes we have about death influence how we live all aspects of our lives. In what ways do your feelings and attitudes about death influence your own lifestyle and experience? (Do you defy death by being a daredevil? Do you deny death by avoiding wakes and funerals? Do you lessen the importance of death by espousing a religious promising eternal life? Do you attempt to accept death by being fatalistic?)

How do these feelings and attitudes about death affect how you currently cope with loss experiences, positively and negatively?

How does your interest in working with dying patients and the bereaved fit in with your issues related to death?

Adapted from Rando TA. Grief, dying, and death: clinical interventions for caregivers. Champaign (IL): Research Press; 1984. p. 9–12; with permission. Copyright 1984 by Therese A. Rando.

---

adolescents feel less isolated by learning what their questions are and answering them concretely. Talking with the adolescent is a sensitive two-way process, where active listening is important—paying attention not only to what the adolescent says, but how they are saying it. Are their facial expressions congruent to the words coming out of

---

Box 2
Your sociocultural, ethnic, and religious/philosophic attitudes toward death

Reflect on your upbringing and socialization. Think about areas such as afterlife; burial rites; expected attitudes of loved ones toward the dying person before and after death; expected attitude of the dying person; expected differences in reaction to death due to age or gender; meaning of death to life; attitude toward caregivers; or attitude toward telling children about death. Then note those attitudes held toward death by your social group, cultural group, ethnic group, and religious/philosophic group.

Which norms, mores, beliefs, sanctions, and attitudes have you internalized about death from these groups?

How do these ideas affect the ways in which you work with the terminally ill and the bereaved, positively and negatively?

Adapted from Rando TA. Grief, dying, and death: clinical interventions for caregivers. Champaign (IL): Research Press; 1984. p. 12–3; with permission. Copyright 1984 by Therese A. Rando.

their mouth? Are they looking away while speaking? Are they telling you they are not worried while complaining of headaches, stomachaches, and sleeplessness? It will be important to be aware of such nonverbal cues as they can provide insight into the adolescents' experiences, thoughts, and feelings about their illness, thus facilitating further communication.

The truth, carefully put, is more helpful than a distortion or an evasion, which could cause a feeling of isolation or be misinterpreted. In a sample of 56 children with cancer, the children who received open information from their parents about their diagnosis and prognosis showed significantly less anxiety and depression.[14] Providing information increases the child's freedom to ask questions and express worries and reduces loneliness, alienation, and isolation.

The usual method of "see one, do one, teach one" may not be an effective way to prepare HCPs to discuss health care planning with youth who have life-limiting illnesses.[15] Many clinicians report a lack of experience or formal training.[16] Fortunately, in many hospitals, adolescents are generally healthy and death is rare. Therefore, ACP conversations may require more formal communication training; there are several programs available such as ComSkil,[17] SPIKES,[18] VitalTalk from the University of Washington (http://vitaltalk.org/),[19] Education in Palliative & End-of-Life Care (EPEC) at Northwestern University's Feinberg School of Medicine (http://www.epec.net/),[20] and Palliative Care Education and Practice (PCEP) at Harvard Medical School (http://www.hms.harvard.edu/pallcare/PCEP/PCEP.htm).[21]

Although open verbal communication is a productive and efficient way to increase patients' and families' understanding and make decisions about ACP, other ancillary services may help as well. Art, music, and play therapy can be used to assist with coping and communication. Child Life or Recreation Therapy Services may be used to introduce medical play and other age-appropriate activities to help explain procedures and gain mastery as well as provide recreation/diversion.

Understand Health Care Provider Barriers

HCPs face many barriers to talking to their patients about ACP, especially when talking about poor prognoses or end-of-life care. Common misconceptions in HCPs about discussing ACP include that talking about end-of-life will make it happen (magical thinking) and that it will increase rates of depression, threaten patients' and families' hope, and reduce rates of survival.[22] In addition to these misconceptions, HCPs may also have reservations due to incomplete knowledge of the patient's prognosis and difficulty handling the emotional nature of the news.[22] However, research has suggested that prognosis *is not necessary* before initiating end-of-life care discussions.[23]

PATIENT AND FAMILY READINESS

After a HCP has explored their own thoughts about death and dying and has learned about communicating with adolescents on this difficult topic, the next step is to assess the patient's readiness for the discussion. Adolescents and their families cope with terminal illness very differently. Productive conversations occur over time and are developmentally appropriate, culturally and religiously sensitive, and tailored to the specific child and family. There may be conflicts across beliefs within the family, between the family and the medical team, and within the medical teams about what information to share, treatments to pursue, and other difficult decisions. This is common and consultations from Psychiatry, Bioethics, and Palliative Care are often available to help clarify and facilitate communication around such conflicts.[24]

What Is Developmentally Appropriate?

Ensuring that the conversations are developmentally appropriate is critical to understanding how to talk to adolescents about death. The adolescent category can span from 12 to 24 years old, which includes individuals with a unique set of experiences in vastly different life stages. This poses a challenge for health care workers not well-versed in the spectrum of normal social, emotional, cognitive, and language skills in adolescent development. An understanding of typical adolescent development is crucial in order to identify emotional and behavioral problems.

VIGNETTE 1

GR is a 15-year-old Hispanic female with a chronic immunodeficiency, recurrent infections and mild developmental delay. She fell behind in school starting in the 5th grade due to missing a lot of school secondary to illness and feeling tired all the time. She receives 1 hour twice a week home schooling to make up her school but at this rate she cannot catch up. Neuropsychological testing shows her full scale IQ to be 70 and her achievement to be at the 3rd grade level. While she has a hard time keeping up with her academic skills, she is friendly and talks readily about the clothes she wants and pop-stars and movies she likes. She is close to her mother who stays with her in the hospital for months at a time. She also has a 27-year-old brother with whom she is close and looks up to who is studying to be a policeman. She feels angry with her father who does not help her mother take care of her or the rest of the family. She reports he is verbally abusive to her, calling her 'lazy' and 'stupid'. She is about the size of a 10-year-old due to her chronic illness.

Psychiatry is consulted initially to evaluate GR for anxiety and depression. She is tired of being in the hospital for several months because they are unable to get her infections under control. Eventually, it is clear, she is failing medically. Despite her "intellectual disability," she is able to answer the question, "if you are too sick, who would you like to make your medical decisions?" She indicates that she wants her mother to make decisions if she is not able to participate. She would also like her brother to help her mother. She does not believe her father will act in her best interest because he has avoided visiting the hospital and has not been active in her home care. She is able to discuss what she is worried about for her mother after she dies.

Understanding of death as a concept

A person's understanding about death includes understanding 4 general concepts: universality, irreversibility, nonfunctionality, and causality.[25] Although every child learns these concepts in the context of their age, developmental stage, and environment, a complete understanding of death in most children generally emerges by 10 years old and current research suggests that much younger children understand concepts of death.[26,27] Living with a serious or terminal illness may cause youth to have an advanced understanding of death.[28] Therefore, knowing that a patient may have a different conceptualization of what death means and understanding the patient's beliefs are very important (**Table 1**).

At different developmental stages, children will experience death as a physical separation or, alternatively, as a punishment that is perhaps temporary. As they get older and understand death is permanent, fear and regression remain common reactions. Adolescents often believe they are immortal despite the evidence before them and may take risks such as nonadherence to medication regimens or try smoking when they know they have cancer. These may be developmentally appropriate risk-taking behaviors, but the stakes are higher when they have a serious or life-threatening illness and pose challenges to themselves and the team caring for them. They often experience hospitalization and dying as a loss of privacy and independence. Denial can be a healthy defense in many cases but becomes dangerous when it interferes with treatment.

Table 1
Children's understanding of death

Concept of Death	Definition	Questions Youth Ask
Universality	All living things die	Does everyone die? Can anyone not die?
Irreversibility	Once dead, dead is forever	Does everyone have to die? How long do you stay dead? Do you/I have to die? What can I/we do to avoid death? When will you die? At any time?
Nonfunctionality	All functions of the body stop	What do you do when you are dead? Do you see? Hear? Smell? Feel?
Causality	What causes death	Why do people die? What caused my pet to die? Can you wish someone dead? When mom said, 'you'll be the death of me one day,' is that why she died?
Afterward	After death	What happens next? Where does the soul go? My spirit? Will I come back to life again? Will I have hair in heaven?

Decision-making of adolescents

The capacity to think abstractly and problem-solving abilities of adolescents are variable as many neurobiological systems mature fully.[29] Increasingly, the treatment choices to be made carry implications for long-term development such as loss of fertility or cognitive abilities and fear of recurrence or second malignancies. In addition, there are 3 main developmental tasks of adolescents:

1. To establish independence from parents/family,
2. To form one's identity, and
3. To create and sustain intimacy with a significant other.

These 3 tasks are often harder to achieve when one is chronically ill. Adolescents wish to be as "normal" as possible, fear rejection, and rely increasingly on peers for their identity, often trying on new and different personas. Being smaller or looking different or being sick and missing out on usual peer activities can disrupt an adolescent's ability to become more independent or closer with peers at a particularly important time in development. Being able to ask for help and cultivate social support is one of the most critical factors in coping with setbacks and later successful transition to adulthood.[30] As seen in Vignette 1, even adolescents with cognitive impairments and mild developmental delay may have sufficient capacity to choose a surrogate medical decision-maker.

A relatively safe place to start when talking with adolescents about their medical decision-making is by asking questions as in **Box 3**, preferably at an outpatient visit when the adolescent is medically stable.

Box 3
Decision-making questions for adolescents

"Has anyone talked with you about what you would like to happen if you become seriously ill in the future?"

"Is there someone you would like to help you make these decisions?"

"Who in your family? Who on your medical team or in the hospital?"

> **Box 4**
> **Questions to assess preferences between monitors and blunters**
>
> "Are you someone who likes to know everything about what's going to happen and when it will happen—the big picture? Or are you someone who likes to know a little bit at a time or, say, just before you need your blood taken, for example?"
>
> "Does it help you to talk about things that are hard or are on your mind or are you someone who wants to work things out alone?"
>
> "What is the hardest thing for you right now?"

Individual personality factors

In addition to identifying where an adolescent is in the developmental understanding of death and dying, it is important to appreciate their personality and preferences. Individuals have their own preferences for how they like to receive information, and each type presents different challenges for health care planning and end-of-life discussions. For example, "monitors" are those individuals who seek detailed information, whereas "blunters" like to avoid anything but the most basic facts.[31] HCPs should ask adolescents how much information they prefer to be given, from whom they prefer to receive information, and whether they prefer information to be provided verbally, in written form, or both ways.

In general, "monitors" will want more medical information, but then may be quite distressed by it and require considerable support with what they learn. "Blunters," while wishing to avoid detailed medical information, may not have sufficient information to make informed decisions. Asking the following questions may help to assess preferences and thus prepare for any challenges (**Box 4**).

Contextual factors

There are vast cultural and ethnic differences in the preferences regarding treatment options, perceptions of death, and discussions about ACP and end-of-life care.[32] Furthermore, religion and spirituality may influence perception of palliative care, coping, and end-of-life decision-making.[33] Although religion and spirituality are often found to serve a protective or supportive role in coping with serious or terminal illness, each adolescent and family will cope differently.[34] It is important to assess whether culture is why parents may be reluctant to communicate to their adolescent the severity of his or her condition. Always ask about each family's basic cultural, ethnic, spiritual, and religious beliefs (**Box 5**).

Language

Fundamental to communication is a shared language. Many HCPs identify language barriers as an obstacle to ACP with adolescents.[35] Always use hospital interpretation services, rather than family or friends who speak the specific language, during ACP.

> **Box 5**
> **Assessing spirituality**
>
> "Can you tell me about your faith or spiritual beliefs?"
>
> "Are there spiritual or religious practices you would like incorporated into your care?"
>
> "Tell me how your family/community feels your adolescent's illness should be handled."

Although a language barrier may not exist per se, patients and families may have vastly different levels of understanding of medical and legal terms or language. It is especially critical to clarify terms when thinking about having discussions with children and their families. Before ACP conversations, concepts of health and death literacy must be assessed.[36] The Plain Language Planner for Palliative Care is a tool to help HCPs recognize and limit their use of medical jargon and thus increase patient health literacy.[37]

Family Adaption: Risk and Resilience Factors

Although ACP should be patient-focused, adolescents are situated within a social and family network that must also be considered. Family factors may influence the timing and manner of ACP conversations. Furthermore, understanding the psychosocial dynamics of the family system is crucial to patient-centered care. One useful tool, the Psychosocial Assessment Tool, assesses factors that place families and caregivers at risk, including structure/resources, family problems, social support, stress reactions, family beliefs, child problems, and sibling problems.[38] These subscales build into the Pediatric Psychosocial Preventative Health Model, where families fall into 1 of 3 levels of overall psychosocial risk—universal, targeted, or clinical/treatment—and limited treatment resources are allocated according to risk level.[38] In a study of 5 different chronic childhood medical conditions, Herzer and colleagues[39] (2010) used the Family Assessment Device to assess family functioning. They found that risk factors include older child age, fewer children in the home, and lower socioeconomic status. Although many factors may contribute to how a family adapts to a chronic or terminal illness (**Table 2**), a family's overall functioning plays a part in the pediatric patient's well-being.[40]

ENGAGING ADOLESCENTS IN ADVANCE CARE PLANNING

ACP refers to the process of HCPs talking about medical decisions in an open, honest, and comfortable manner, making themselves available to the adolescent and their families for an ongoing discussion around these issues. These conversations may not always be planned or necessarily lengthy once the relationship around and permission to talk about these topics is established early as safe topics to bring up. Otherwise, such conversations may not occur at all or happen too late when the adolescent is too ill to participate in a meaningful way.

Table 2
Factors affecting family adaptation

Predictors of Positive Family Adaptation	Predictors of Family and Caregiver Risk
• Family cohesion and flexibility	• Lone parenting with limited social support
• Ability to reorganize and balance demands of the illness with family needs and responsibilities	• Estranged or chronically conflicted relationships
	• Marital discord
• Clear family boundaries	• Preexisting medical and/or psychiatric problems
• Open and effective communication	• Socioeconomic vulnerabilities (unemployment, transportation, insurance)
• Active coping	• Limited access to support
• Strong spiritual belief system	• Cultural and language barriers, rigid religious belief system
• Ability to seek social support from extended family, church, work place, community	• Lack of consensus re: research, aggressive care
	• Climate of secrecy

In 2004, Himelstein and colleagues[41] outlined 4 specific components to what is now referred to as ACP. First, there is identification of the decision-makers, including the adolescent; second, clarification of the patients' and parents' understanding of the illness and prognosis; third, establishment of care goals as curative, uncertain, or comfort care; and fourth, joint decision-making regarding use or nonuse of life-sustaining medical interventions such as mechanical ventilation, intravenous hydration, or phase I chemotherapy. Complicated and serious decisions such as these clearly take time and may evolve over the course of an illness as well.

Creating an Advance Care Planning Document

Voicing My CHOiCES™
Initial research with 52 adolescent and young adults (AYAs), aged 16 to 28 years, who were living with a life-threatening illness, such as human immunodeficiency virus infection or recurrent or metastatic cancer, showed that these AYA, although they might find it stressful, wanted to be able to participate in choosing the kind of medical treatment they wanted as well as to express their end-of-life wishes.[42] Following this research, further adaptation of Five Wishes, an adult ACP guide, resulted in the development of *Voicing My CHOiCES™: An Advanced Care Planning Guide for Adolescents & Young Adults*.[43–45] The document allows patients to reflect on and record the following:

1. The kind of medical treatment they want and do not want,
2. How they would like to be cared for,
3. Information for their family and friends to know, and
4. How they would like to be remembered.

Voicing My CHOiCES™ became available to the public in November 2012. Moreover, *Voicing My CHOiCES™* is written so HCPs can read parts of it verbatim to AYA in order to be more comfortable with end-of-life language. Each topic within the document can be presented, by a trusted medical team member, as a separate module starting with the sections addressing comfort or support. The modules do not have to be completed all in one sitting and should be tailored to the patients' concerns at the time. Additional specific language and timing on how to initiate these difficult conversations using *Voicing My CHOiCES™* are available.[46] Since 2012, new Internet sites are available online to facilitate end-of-life conversations, although none are targeted to AYA (http://deathcafe.com/; http://deathoverdinner.org/; http://theconversationproject.org/; www.joincake.com/welcome/; www.dyingmatters.org/; www.begintheconversation.org/).

These documents serve as a guidepost for the adolescent's desires for quality of life and may change over time as a disease progresses and additional treatments are unsuccessful. They are not legal documents for adolescents younger than 18 years and are mutable should the adolescent make new decisions as they gain a better understanding of their impending mortality.

Family-centered Advance Care Planning (FACE) intervention
Maureen Lyon and colleagues[47] at Children's National Health System developed an intervention for adolescents with chronic or terminal medical illness, consisting of a disease-specific ACP interview and completion of an advance directive. Although patients reported that these discussions prompted feelings of sadness, the patients and families involved in the intervention found it useful and helpful.[48] There may be significant areas of discordance between

youth and their families when considering timing of end-of-life medical de-cisions discussions, but in a randomized controlled trial of the ACP intervention versus sham intervention, there were higher rates of concordance between adolescent patients and their families following the pediatric ACP intervention.[49,50]

ACP research is emerging to include other medical conditions as well, such as congenital heart disease, cystic fibrosis, muscular dystrophy and other neuromuscular diseases, and youth on long-term assisted ventilation.[51–54] The literature consistently demonstrates the need for ACP for youth with these serious medical conditions. How-ever, further research is needed to understand the unique challenges that each pop-ulation confronts and to develop valid interventions to foster these important discussions.

VIGNETTE 2

LW is an 18-year-old with relapsed acute lymphocytic leukemia who had 2 failed bone marrow transplants and is admitted for experimental chemotherapy. He is legally allowed to make his own decisions, but he feels unprepared to do so. His parents have supported him throughout and do not want to talk about the possibility of a negative outcome.

Parents are willing to have LW complete an advance care document, but they do not want to be the ones to bring it up.

In his advance care plan, LW was able to tell the health care worker that he wanted a celebra-tion of his life with a pizza party and that he wished to be buried wearing his favorite hockey team's cap.

A CONVERSATION ABOUT ADVANCE CARE PLANNING INCLUDING END-OF-LIFE WISHES
When?

It is not easy to know when is best to initiate ACP conversations with patients and families. It requires a balancing act between the adolescent's readiness and that of their family's and, separately, the HCP's readiness. If an HCP were to ask the following questions (**Box 6**) and the answer is "no" to each, then it might be time to consider initiating an ACP discussion.[55] It is also helpful to check to see if the adolescent is prepared to open an end-of-life discussion, which can be probed us-ing a readiness assessment by asking adolescents whether end-of-life conversa-tions would be helpful or upsetting, and if they feel comfortable discussing preferences when treatment options become limited.[42,44,46]

Critical to the success of end-of-life discussions is identifying the adolescent's personal beliefs, values, and goals, particularly as they relate to their quality of life. It is difficult to initiate an ACP discussion at the time of diagnosis or relapse because the adolescent and their family often does not hear or process much beyond the immediate bad news. While during hospitalization is a convenient time for HCPs to initiate ACP discussions, this time may not be opportune because the adolescent is likely to be regressed, stressed, and in a more dependent mode. Therefore, often the ideal time is during a routine outpatient visit when the adolescent is medically and emotionally stable. Understanding that a prognosis *is not necessary* before initiating such discussions is important.[23] Developing a consistent message around openness to talking about the adolescent's wishes

---

Box 6
Questions to ask HCP to gauge readiness to discuss advance care planning

Would you be surprised if this adolescent died prematurely due to a life-limiting illness?

Would you be surprised if this adolescent died within a year?

Would you be surprised if this adolescent died during this episode of care?

Do you know what the adolescent's and family's wishes are for the end-of-life?

From Brook L, et al. A Plan for Living and a Plan for Dying: Advanced Care Planning for Children. Arch Dis Child 2008; 93 (suppl): A61-6; with permission.

---

and ambitions at regular intervals that an HCP can implement routinely may be helpful.

HCPs should demonstrate that communicating about end-of-life informs the adolescent and their family of the medical team's goal to respect individual wishes and affirm the role of surrogate decision-making. If parents tell the medical team not to give an adolescent any medical information, it is important to review thoroughly the family history and religious, spiritual, or cultural beliefs. Further exploration and discussion with parents regarding their discomfort and reluctance about open communication with their adolescent can be helpful. In some cultures where disclosure and transparency are not the norm, the team may have to respect the family's wishes against their personal wishes. The medical team should explain that if an adolescent asks a question that the team is constrained from answering, the adolescent will be told that their parents have asked them not to answer that question and that the adolescent should discuss it with the parents. In this situation, the team may consider discussions with other family members (with parental and patient permission) and religious counselors of the same faith, or request for an ethics consultation.

Sometimes an adolescent will be ready to stop pursing treatment after a long course of illness. It may be appropriate to have a psychiatric consultation when the adolescent reports a desire to stop the treatment, that they are "tired", or that they "don't care anymore," for example, to rule out any depression or anxiety disorder that may respond to treatment. In contrast, the psychiatry consultant may point out the adolescent has no psychiatric disorder, has capacity for medical decision-making, and should be supported in their wishes.

VIGNETTE 3

DM is a 16-year-old male who was first diagnosed with osteosarcoma when he was 12 years old. After 5 years of treatment with chemotherapy, surgical resection of metastatic lung nodules on 2 separate occasions, and a third relapse of multiple metastatic pulmonary and bony lesions, DM reports he is "tired" of treatments. He has spent a significant part of the past 5 years in the hospital. His primary caretaker is his maternal grandfather. Psychiatry is consulted to evaluate for depression, and the consultant determines that the DM is not depressed and has capacity to make medical decisions.

DM participates in his medical decision-making and indicates he wants his grandfather to make his medical decisions when he is not able. He trusts his grandfather knows what he wants. DM wants intubation if he has something that can be treated but he does not want to be kept alive if there is no chance of his improving to have significant quality of life.

Who?

Although ACP conversations should be patient-centered and focused on the wishes of the adolescent, there are often several other important individuals and medical services that may need to be included. Ask about who else is involved in the care of the patient and family (eg, pediatric palliative care service, religious or spiritual services, a special physical therapist, a psychologist or consultation psychiatrist etc.).[56] If working together with a trusted medical team member or other service team on *Voicing My CHOiCES*™, adolescents may complete some sections independently, but it is highly recommended that they work alongside a HCP, particularly when making decisions about life support treatments.

What?

Despite being young, adolescents with terminal or life-threatening illness do think about what will happen after their death, and they are able to make concrete decisions about their preferences. When working with an advanced care planning document, adolescents and young adults demonstrate greater interest in discussing and documenting preferences about how they will be treated and remembered, rather than medical or legal technicalities.[42] As part of the ACP, adolescents can voice preferences about type of service (funeral, memorial service, or celebration of life), treatment of their body (burial, cremation, organ donor, donation to science, autopsy), and publicity (open or closed casket).[43] They can make decisions about the arrangements of the service (clothing, food, music, readings), the distribution of their belongings, and request future celebrations in their memory.[43] Allowing these decisions to be made by participating adolescents serves to empower and respect them.

SUMMARY

Talking with adolescents about death and dying is a challenging but powerful and rewarding experience. During the process, most HCPs learn, not only about themselves, but also about the resilience and fortitude that these youths who are coping with severe illnesses and difficult circumstances have to teach us. Open communication can alleviate anxiety and distress by allowing adolescents the ability to express their preferences and helping parents and HCPs make informed decisions while potentially improving the adolescent's quality of life.

REFERENCES

1. Perkins HS. Controlling death: the false promise of advance directives. Ann Intern Med 2007;147(1):51–7.

2. American Academy of Pediatrics. Committee on Bioethics and Committee on Hospital Care. Palliative care for children. Pediatrics 2000;106:351–7.

3. When children die: improving palliative and end-of-life care for children and their families. The National Academies Press; 2003.

4. World Health Organization. Persisting pain in children package: WHO guidelines on the pharmacological treatment of persisting pain in children with medical illnesses. Geneva (Switzerland): World Health Organization; 2012. Available at: http://www.who.int/iris/handle/10665/44540.

5. End of life care for infants, children and young people with life limiting conditions: summary of NICE guidance. BMJ 2016;355. https://doi.org/10.1136/bmj.i6385.

6. Waechter EH. Children's awareness of fatal illness. Am J Nurs 1971;71(6): 1168–72.
7. Bluebond-Langner M. The private worlds of dying children. Princeton (NJ): Princeton U.P; 1980.
8. Kreicbergs U, Valdimarsdóttir U, Onelöv E, et al. Talking about death with children who have severe malignant disease. N Engl J Med 2004;351(12):1175–86.
9. Freyer DR. Care of the dying adolescent. Pediatrics 2004;113:381–8.
10. Hurwitz C, Duncan J, Wolfe J. Caring for the child with cancer at the close of life. JAMA 2004;2992(17):2141–9.
11. Rando TA. Grief, dying, and death: clinical interventions for caregivers. Champaign (IL): Research Press; 1984.
12. Schonfeld DJ, Demaria T, American Academy of Pediatrics, Committee on Psychosocial Aspects of Child and Family Health, Disaster Preparedness Advisory Council. Supporting the grieving child and family. Pediatrics 2016. https://doi.org/10.1542/peds.2016-2147.
13. Breyer J. Talking to children and adolescents. In: Wiener L, Pao M, Kazak A, et al, editors. Quick reference for pediatric oncology clinicians: the psychiatric and psychological dimensions of pediatric cancer symptom management. 2nd edition. Oxford (England): Oxford University Press; 2014.
14. Last BF, van Veldhuizen AM. Information about diagnosis and prognosis related to anxiety and depression in children with cancer aged 8-16 years. Eur J Cancer 1996;32(2):290–4.
15. Feraco AM, Brand SR, Mack JW, et al. Communication skills training in pediatric oncology: moving beyond role modeling. Pediatr Blood Cancer 2016. https://doi.org/10.1002/pbc.25918.
16. Sanderson A, Hall AM, Wolfe J. Advance care discussions: pediatric clinician preparedness and practices. J Pain Symptom Manage 2016;51(3):520–8.
17. Kissane DW, Bylund CL, Banerjee SC, et al. Communication skills training for oncology professionals. J Clin Oncol 2012;30:1242–7.
18. Baile WF, Buckman R, Lenzi R, et al. SPIKES—a six-step protocol for delivering bad news: application to the patient with cancer. Oncologist 2000;5:302–11.
19. VitalTalk. (n.d.). Available at: http://vitaltalk.org/. Accessed April 16, 2018.
20. Education in palliative and end-of-life care. (n.d.). Available at: http://www.epec.net/. Accessed April 16, 2018.
21. Multidisciplinary training for professionals. (n.d.). Available at: http://www.hms.harvard.edu/pallcare/PCEP/PCEP.htm, Accessed April 16, 2018.
22. Mack JW, Smith TJ. Reasons why physicians do not have discussions about poor prognosis, why it matters, and what can be improved. J Clin Oncol 2012;30(22): 2715–7.
23. Waldman E, Wolfe J. Palliative care for children with cancer. Nat Rev Clin Oncol 2013;10(2):100–7.
24. Muriel AC, Wolfe J, Block SD. Pediatric palliative care and child psychiatry: a model for enhancing practice and collaboration. J Palliat Med 2016;19(10): 1032–8.
25. Kenyon BL. Current research in children's conceptions of death: a critical review. Omega 2001;43:63–91.
26. Bates AT, Kearney JA. Understanding death with limited experience in life: dying children's and adolescents' understanding of their own terminal illness and death. Curr Opin Support Palliat Care 2015;9(1):40–5.

27. Luby J, Belden A, Sullivan J, et al. Shame and guilt in preschool depression: evidence for elevations in self-conscious emotions in depression as early as age 3. J Child Psychol Psychiatry 2009;50(9):1156–66.

28. Jay SM, Green V, Johnson S, et al. Differences in death concepts between children with cancer and physically healthy children. J Clin Child Psychol 1987;16: 301–6.

29. Mills KL, Goddings AL, Clasen LS, et al. The developmental mismatch in structural brain maturation during adolescence. Dev Neurosci 2014;36(3–4):147–60.

30. Pao M. Conceptualization of success in young adulthood. Child Adolesc Psychiatr Clin N Am 2017;26(2):191–8.

31. Miller SM. Monitoring and blunting: validation of a questionnaire to assess styles of information seeking under threat. J Pers Soc Psychol 1987;52(2):345–53.

32. Ohr S, Jeong S, Saul P. Cultural and religious beliefs and values, and their impact on preferences for end-of-life care among four ethnic groups of community-dwelling older persons. J Clin Nurs 2017;26(11–12):1681–9.

33. Steinberg SM. Cultural and religious aspects of palliative care. Int J Crit Illn Inj Sci 2011;1(2):154–6.

34. López-Sierra HE, Rodríguez-Sánchez J. The supportive roles of religion and spirituality in end-of-life and palliative care of patients with cancer in a culturally diverse context: a literature review. Curr Opin Support Palliat Care 2015;9(1): 87–95.

35. Davies B1, Sehring SA, Partridge JC, et al. Barriers to palliative care for children: perceptions of pediatric health care providers. Pediatrics 2008;121(2):282–8.

36. Hayes B, Fabri AM, Coperchini M, et al. Health and death literacy and cultural diversity: insights from hospital-employed interpreters. BMJ Support Palliat Care 2017. https://doi.org/10.1136/bmjspcare-2016-001225.

37. Wittenberg E, Goldsmith J, Ferrell B, et al. Enhancing communication related to symptom management through plain language. J Pain Symptom Manage 2015; 50(5):707–11.

38. Kazak AE, Schneider S, Didonato S, et al. Family psychosocial risk screening guided by the pediatric psychosocial preventative health model (PPPHM) using the psychosocial assessment tool (PAT). Acta Oncol 2015;54(5):574–80.

39. Herzer M, Godiwala N, Hommel KA, et al. Family functioning in the context of pediatric chronic conditions. J Dev Behav Pediatr 2010;31(1):26.

40. Leeman J, Crandell JL, Lee A, et al. Family functioning and the well-being of children with chronic conditions: a meta-analysis. Res Nurs Health 2016;39(4): 229–43.

41. Himelstein BP, Hilden JM, Morstad Boldt A, et al. Pediatric palliative care. N Engl J Med 2004;350:1752–62.

42. Wiener L, Ballard E, Brennan T, et al. How I wish to be remembered: the use of an advance care planning document in adolescent and young adult populations. J Palliat Med 2008;11(10):1309–13.

43. Five wishes. Aging with Dignity; 2018. Available at: www.agingwithdignity.org/.

44. Wiener L, Zadeh S, Battles H, et al. Allowing adolescents and young adults to plan their end-of-life care. Pediatrics 2012. https://doi.org/10.1542/peds.2012-0663.

45. Wiener L, Zadeh S, Wexler L, et al. When silence is not golden: engaging adolescents and young adults in discussions around end-of-life care. Pediatr Blood Cancer 2013;60:715–8.

46. Zadeh S, Pao M, Wiener L. Opening end-of-life discussions: how to introduce using voicing my choices, an advance care planning guide for adolescents and young adults. Palliat Support Care 2015;13(3):591–9.

47. Kimmel AL, Wang J, Scott RK, et al. Family centered (FACE) advance care planning: study design and methods for a patient-centered communication and decision-making intervention for patients with HIV/AIDS and their surrogate decision-makers. Contemp Clin Trials 2015;43:172–8.

48. Dallas RH, Kimmel A, Wilkins ML, et al. Acceptability of family-centered advanced care planning for adolescents with HIV. Pediatrics 2016;138(6) [pii: e20161854].

49. Lyon ME, Dallas RH, Garvie PA, et al. Paediatric advance care planning survey: a cross-sectional examination of congruence and discordance between adolescents with HIV/AIDS and their families. BMJ Support Palliat Care 2017. https://doi.org/10.1136/bmjspcare-2016-001224.

50. Lyon ME, D'Angelo LJ, Dallas RH, et al. A randomized clinical trial of adolescents with HIV/AIDS: pediatric advance care planning. AIDS Care 2017;29(10): 1287–96.

51. Tobler D, Greutmann M, Colman JM, et al. Knowledge of and preference for advance care planning by adults with congenital heart disease. Am J Cardiol 2012;109(12):1797–800.

52. Kazmerski TM, Weiner DJ, Matisko J, et al. Advance care planning in adolescents with cystic fibrosis: a quality improvement project. Pediatr Pulmonol 2016;51(12): 1304–10.

53. Hiscock A, Kuhn I, Barclay S. Advance care discussions with young people affected by life-limiting neuromuscular diseases: a systematic literature review and narrative synthesis. Neuromuscul Disord 2017. https://doi.org/10.1016/j.nmd.2016.11.011.

54. Edwards JD, Kun SS, Graham RJ, et al. End-of-life discussions and advance care planning for children on long-term assisted ventilation with life-limiting conditions. J Palliat Care 2012;28(1):21–7.

55. Brook L, et al. A plan for living and a plan for dying: advanced care planning for children. Arch Dis Child 2008;93(suppl):A61–6.

56. Buxton D. Child and adolescent psychiatry and palliative care. J Am Acad Child Adolesc Psychiatry 2015;54:791–2.

Supporting Children and Families at a Child's End of Life

Pediatric Palliative Care Pearls of Anticipatory Guidance for Families

Bethany Lockwood, MD[a],*, Lisa Humphrey, MD[b]

KEYWORDS

• End of life • Palliative • Pediatrics • Hospice • Mental health provider

KEY POINTS

• Use the child's signs and symptoms as a guide to prognostication.
• Continue to empower the parental role, as this is a unique gift only they can offer.
• Help prepare patients and families for what they may see, hear, and experience during the dying process.

INTRODUCTION

A child's death has been described as the *ultimate loss*,[1] and preparing for this often seems unnatural and illogical. Mercifully, pediatric deaths are relatively uncommon; however, given this rarity, health care providers are often unfamiliar and uncomfortable with supporting the dying child. Pediatric death occurs under different circumstances, ranging from acutely in the neonatal period to perhaps expectedly as a young adult from a congenital life-limiting disease, thus requiring different skill sets for preparation and anticipatory grieving for families.[2] This article seeks to provide clinical pearls from pediatric palliative care providers to help patients and families process and prepare for a child's death.

Disclosure Statement: Neither L. Humphrey nor B. Lockwood have any financial or other affiliations to disclose at this time.
[a] Division of Palliative Medicine, The Ohio State University College of Medicine, McCampbell Hall, 5th Floor, 1581 Dodd Drive, Columbus, OH 43210, USA; [b] Hospice and Palliative Medicine, Nationwide Children's Hospital, The Ohio State University College of Medicine, 700 Children's Drive, A1055, Columbus, OH 43205, USA
* Corresponding author.
E-mail address: Bethany.Lockwood@osumc.edu

EDUCATING PATIENTS AND FAMILIES ABOUT PALLIATIVE CARE

Case: Your patient, Daniel, a 21-year-old with hypoplastic left heart syndrome status post a Fontan procedure, now has severe ventricular dysfunction and is being considered for heart transplantation. The primary team consults palliative care. You have known this patient for multiple years due to his depression and anxiety. He asks to speak to you because he is worried that "the death doctors are coming to talk me out of a heart transplant."

Pediatric palliative care is the medical specialty that addresses the many stressors experienced by pediatric and young adult patients with life-threatening conditions. It addresses physical symptoms (eg, pain, nausea, insomnia), spiritual, and psychosocial stressors that can negatively impact quality of life. Additionally, palliative care seeks to ensure that the patient and caregivers have maximal comprehension of their health issues and medical choices, and that the health care team understands the patient's hopes and seeks to align patient goals with medical interventions as able. There can be discordance between hopes and what medicine can offer. In these cases, palliative care partners with the patient, family, and the health care team for optimal communication and decision making. At times, patients may transition to hospice care, a specific type of palliative care that provides end-of-life care for the dying patient that still attends to the many domains of care, including physical, psychological, social, spiritual, and cultural.

ACCEPTING THE DEATH OF A CHILD

Case: Susie is a 16-year-old girl with high-risk acute myelogenous leukemia who received stem cell transplantation 3 weeks ago. Her single mother sits vigilant at Susie's bedside in the pediatric intensive care unit. She was transferred 1 week ago due to renal and respiratory failure prompting need for continuous dialysis, intubation, and mechanical ventilation. Susie has not shown signs of clinical improvement. You have been consulted to provide support and help her mother "comprehend and accept" her daughter's mortality risk.

Letting go of the goal for cure and moving toward hope for a comfortable death is an extremely challenging transition for patients, families, and health care providers. Caregivers may have difficulty understanding why previously effective therapies are no longer beneficial. They also struggle with the emotions of failing their child. As providers, you can help guide families through this transition from *life preservation*, preventing the loss and prolonging the life of their child, to *letting go*, recognizing the inevitable death and shift in focus to the child's needs and well-being.[3]

There are a number of factors that influence parental readiness for their child's death. The perspective of *letting go* is supported by certainty that the child cannot be cured, perception of suffering with visible symptom burden, an ability to separate their own needs from their child's, and the ability to parent meaningfully.[3] Some caregivers can transition to death acceptance solely through these exposures and capacities; others can with additional clinical support. There are also caregivers who may never be able to transition from a goal of cure to a goal of comfort.

Each type of caregiver requires a different supportive approach. The caregiver who independently transitions will benefit from reassurance that there is emotional and practical reinforcement from the health care team. For those who transition with support, techniques such as motivational interviewing can be transformational. Clinician reassurance that a transition from a goal of cure to a goal of comfort is the action of a loving, good parent is also paramount.[4] Finally, those parents who cannot pivot from curative intent to death acceptance need clinicians who acknowledge their unwavering love and hope, but also ones that can bear the mantle of decision making and be more forthright in what constitutes a reasonable and respectful care plan. This may include nonescalation or discontinuation of therapies whose burdens vastly outweigh their benefit. Mental health professionals play a key role in guiding and supporting their health care colleagues toward such action.

ADVANCED CARE PLANNING

Case: You have been working with a mother of a 6-year-old girl, Lacy, with a progressive mitochondrial disorder. Mom recognizes her daughter's functional decline and articulates sadness that her daughter is no longer able to express joy. Additionally, the girl is frequently hospitalized for issues secondary to her decline, such as aspiration pneumonia and refractory seizures. Recently a physician spoke to mom about code status. Mom asks you, "Why would a doctor ask me that? Why wouldn't I wish to do everything for my child?"

Advanced care planning is an umbrella term that encapsulates end-of-life wishes and decisions. It includes concepts such as health care power of attorney designation, identifying the desired location of death, code status, and legacy work. When done well, all aspects of advanced care planning are equally emphasized and presented in a methodical process at a pace set by the decision maker and not the health care provider.

Advanced Care Planning Tools

Many providers feel underprepared or unskilled to discuss these advance care planning topics. However, there are many resources to help prepare for and guide one through the conversation. Often the patient's social worker is a great resource in providing and facilitating advance care planning documents. Advanced care planning workbooks also exist to help guide you. For example, Aging with Dignity, a nonprofit organization that advocates for quality care at the end of life has developed guide books for all ages to help with this conversation.[5] *My Wishes*, for school-aged children and *Voicing My Choices*, for adolescents and young adults, use developmentally appropriate language and themes to allow children facing serious illness to express and share their preferences for how they want to be cared for and remembered.[5] Although these are not legal documents, they do help to introduce this very important conversation. For adults, Aging with Dignity uses *Five Wishes*, which is a legal advanced care planning document in 42 states, offered in 28 languages, and seeks to be more user friendly than many state-sponsored documents.[5] In states in which *Five Wishes* is not a recognized legal document, it can still be completed first to facilitate ease of completing the state-issued document.

Finally, there are several game-based tools to assist with pediatric and young adult advanced care planning. One example is the card game *Go Wish*, produced by the Coda Alliance, which offers an interactive, game-oriented way to think and talk about what is important in the face of serious illness.[6] This uses 36 cards with a variety of things people often say are important when they are very sick or dying (eg, to have family with me, to be free from pain, to be at peace with God). The cards include items related to how people want to be treated, who they want nearby, where they want to be, and what matters most.[6] It can be completed individually by the patient but it is best to have the patient partner with a health care provider who is skilled in translating the preferred cards into an advanced care plan.

Advanced Care Planning Concepts

In addition to such resources, health care providers need to be armed with how to discuss the logistics embedded within end-of-life care planning. The most recognized of these tasks is code status consideration. Unfortunately, health care providers often emphasize code status decisions over other aspects of advanced care planning. This has several consequences. First, this act elevates cardiopulmonary resuscitation (CPR) consideration above other medical decisions at the risk of lending it mythical powers. We often do not adequately discuss the negative outcomes of CPR or the high rates of mortality in medically fragile patients despite CPR being enacted. Many medical providers also do not give their medical opinion regarding its utility; rather, they offer it up as a choice. As a result, parents often internalize the conversation as "save your child versus let your child die." Second, families may cope through denial and perceive code status consideration as a theoretic conversation that does not require engagement. This can stress health care providers who seek code status clarity, and lead to conflict with families. It also can lead to disengagement by patients or caregivers, thereby inhibiting conversations about other aspects of advanced care planning.

To avoid such outcomes, the initial work in advanced care planning should focus on legacy work and aspirations that a patient or family may have. These are equally important in preparing for a child's death. Understanding what the child or young adult and his or her family values the most can assist with achieving certain goals before death and also opens the conversation to discuss the child's legacy and how he or she hopes to be remembered.

After these are determined, identifying the desired location of death should be explored. Locations can include the home, hospital, long-term care facilities, or sometimes an inpatient hospice facility. There are important things to consider about each location, and hospice services often can be provided in all of these settings. Some families may desire their child to be at home, surrounded by familiarity and the comfort of friends and family, as the hospital can often feel like a medicalized sterile environment. It is important to consider who may also be in the home during this experience, including siblings and pets and how this may influence decision making and planned supports. Other families cannot conceive of a home death, and seek to have their child die in the hospital or at a hospice house. Hospice houses are an aspect of the hospice benefit that provides continuous access to medical support for refractory symptoms that cannot be controlled in the home. Although there are very few pediatric hospice houses in the United States, many adult hospice programs will assist children and often will do so even in the absence of refractory symptomatology. Many families who do not wish for a home death often prefer an inpatient death on the unit that frequently cared for their child during hospitalizations. They appreciate the familiarity of the staff and often identify them as primary supports. When supporting an inpatient death, it is important to ensure that medicalization (eg, laboratory draws, vital sign checks) are minimized or avoided so as to allow the focus to remain on the family unit and providing comfort to the child.

The final aspect of advanced care planning is code status consideration. Code status is best discussed when there is recognition by the family that their child is "tired," "losing the battle," or whatever verbiage a caregiver uses to identify that death is a possibility. Such identification by the caregiver signals that the once theoretic consideration of CPR has become a necessary consideration. Still, it is a complex conversation to navigate and the risk of a caregiver feeling the need to "do something" is strong, even if it contradicts a caregiver's stated goal of care. For example, a parent may not want a child to suffer and can even acknowledge that chest compressions can physically hurt, but feel driven to seek CPR at end of life to avoid the sensation of giving up. To counteract this, it is best to acknowledge the desire to do no harm, to reframe the decision to not pursue CPR as a loving decision that avoids suffering and to provide your medical advice that it is not an indicated medical intervention, as it often does not provide the desired healing that families hope for.

ANTICIPATORY GUIDANCE

Case: You recently engaged in advanced care planning with a 19-year-old young man, Joey, with cystic fibrosis, using the guide *Voicing My Choices*. Your team social worker is acquiring the necessary state-approved documents for his completion. He has had multiple hospitalizations for recurrent multidrug-resistant infections, ongoing symptoms of dyspnea, and renal failure related to nephrotoxic antibiotics, and the team shares that he is not a lung transplant candidate. Just as you initiated end-of-life preparation with advanced care planning, you now have an opportunity to provide anticipatory guidance for him and his family as to what else lies ahead.

As discussed with advanced care planning, preparing families for the death experience is paramount. Mental health providers can play an integral part in preparing a family for what they will see, hear, and experience as death approaches. Arming loved ones with such knowledge normalizes the dying process, thereby providing them with reassurance as they witness changes. This also can help families anticipate how much time they may have with their child to allow for last wishes, memory making, and legacy work.

PROGNOSTICATION

Health care providers are often faced with the question: How long does my child have? Prognostication is one of the most wanted answers for patients and families and yet one of the most difficult tasks for providers. Accuracy increases both with clinical experience and as we get closer to the time of death, but often decreases with longer durations of the provider-patient-family relationship.[7,8] Such overestimating and underestimating life expectancy can create anxiety for the family and even distrust of the provider. Thus, it is preferred to give ranges of predicted time to death, such as days to weeks or hours to days. Additionally, relying on the patient's signs and symptoms can assist in selecting the most reliable time frame, as outlined in **Table 1**.[9]

Despite these guidelines, accurate prognostication can remain elusive. Families seek this knowledge to emotionally prepare; however, it is better to reframe this question toward the emotional journey needed to prepare for their child's death. Consider these 4 end-of-life stages described by parents: becoming aware of the inevitable death, making the child's life enjoyable, managing the change for the worse, and being with the dying child.[10] The essence of these end-of-life phases are often better characterized as coping with loss rather than the acceptance of death.[10] Palliative care teams and mental health providers can provide crucial support in identifying and supporting these stages to optimize a caregiver's ability to prepare for their child's death. Providers also can use this prognostication tool

Table 1
Signs and symptoms close to death

	Months	Weeks	Long Days	Short Days	Hours
Physical signs and symptoms					
Activity	Normal as is developmentally appropriate	Weakness, fatigue, partial care	Continued weakness, fatigue, more care needs	Extreme weakness, total care	No muscle tone, minimal to no voluntary movements
Nutrition and hydration	Normal to some weight loss and changes in food preferences	↓ Intake, weight loss (>10%)	↓ Intake, dehydration, dysphagia	Continued dysphagia, dehydration, dry mouth	No oral intake
Elimination	Normal as is developmentally appropriate	Diarrhea, constipation, urinary retention	Bowel/bladder incontinence, concentrated urine	Bowel/bladder incontinence	No urine, bowel incontinence
Pain	Typical for disease state	May be ↑	↑ Total pain	Possible pain	↑ or ↓
Skin	Normal	Increased fragility, injuries	Breakdown and bedsores	Color changes, including pallor, cyanosis	Mottling, ashen, cyanotic distal extremities, livedo reticularis
Sleep	Normal to some sleep disruption	↑ Sleep often >50% daytime in bed	Mostly in bed, restlessness	↑ Sleeping	Nearly constant sleep
Eyes	Normal	Dull appearance	Dull, cloudy, appear distant	Glazed, sunken, unable to close eyes, bloodshot	Glazed fixed stare, partly open, lack of pupillary change
Respirations	Normal for disease state (eg, BPD, CHD)	Some dyspnea, hypoxia	Variable: shallow vs deeper and labored	Increased congestion, "death rattle," Cheyne-Stokes	Prolonged periods of apnea, continued death rattle, Cheyne-Stokes, mouth open

Neurologic	Normal for disease state (eg, HIE, CP)	Normal for disease state	Irritability, agitation, seizures, twitching, delirium	Increased agitation, lack of purposeful movements, hallucinations, delirium	Terminal delirium, often unarousable, may have mysterious "rally"
Edema	None to some edema	↑ Distension and edema	Continued distension and edema	↑ Or ↓ edema	↓ Edema
Psychological signs and symptoms in older children and adolescents					
Emotions	Maintain sense of self	Fear of falling asleep, ↑ anxiety	↑ Fear and uncertainty	Improving peacefulness, fear of being alone	Peacefulness
Facing reality	Denial or acceptance, create "bucket list"	Wants to know what to expect	Acceptance, saying goodbyes	"I'm dying"	Acceptance, goodbyes
Social markers in older children and adolescents					
Interactions	Normal to increased	Withdrawn, depression	Withdrawn	Increasingly withdrawn	Inability to express self
Spiritual markers in older children and adolescents					
	Thoughts about funeral	Dreams of dead/spiritual figures	Continued dreams	May see people who are dead	Performance of spiritual rituals
Family markers					
	Special trips, events as family	Memory making, legacy work	Anticipatory grieving	May feel guilt, ready for patient to die	Gives permission to die, letting go

Abbreviations: ↑, increase; ↓, decrease; BPD, bronchopulmonary dysplasia; CHD, congenital heart disease; CP, cerebral palsy; HIE, hypoxic ischemic encephalopathy.

to assist children and families to reach some of their aspirations related to advanced care planning, as previously discussed. This further emphasizes the importance of discussing legacy work and location of death, so that the medical team can best support the patient and family to meet their goals in the expected time remaining.

SYMPTOMS AT THE END OF LIFE

After facilitating acceptance and estimating prognostication, health care providers should next prepare caregivers for the signs and symptoms they will witness. It is estimated that children may experience 7 to 10 symptoms requiring management at the end of life. There are a number of studies that have explored the most common and distressing symptoms for children at the end of life, with a focus on the pediatric cancer population. Although symptoms may vary based on age and underlying disease process, 4 of the commonly reported symptoms by patients and families are fatigue, pain, dyspnea, and poor appetite.[11,12] Some studies have addressed an even greater number of symptoms, which also included changes in behavior, appearance, sleep pattern, bowel and bladder, and temperature.[13] And even further studies have found a higher mean symptom burden of 11 symptoms, with lack of energy, drowsiness, skin changes, irritability, pain, swelling of extremities, and dry mouth occurring at high prevalence.[14]

Most of the concerning symptoms, including pain, decrease between the week of death to the day of death, while breathing changes may increase.[13] Similarly, studies demonstrate the level of patient comfort improves as the dying process progresses: in the last week of life 64.0%, last day 76.6%, and last hour 93.4% of children were always or usually comfortable.[14] A follow-up evaluation further reviewed descriptive factors that distinguished symptoms of most concern from those not of most concern. Of note, 1 of the 5 factors unique to the category of symptoms NOT of most concern included symptoms for which the parent felt adequately prepared for.[15] This again emphasizes the importance and value of anticipatory guidance for families.

USE YOUR SENSES: WHAT YOU MIGHT EXPERIENCE AS A CAREGIVER FOR A DYING CHILD

> Case: You have been working extensively with the family of Bobby, a 5-year-old boy with a progressive neurodegenerative disease. He was admitted for seizure management that ultimately proved to be refractory to multiple antiepileptic agents. He is at great risk for death by respiratory failure due to frequent and protracted apneas. One day prior, the parents decided not to pursue CPR if Bobby decompensates. Today, they struggle with what his death will be like and they begin peppering you with questions.

How a child dies impacts a parent's ability to cope with this devastating loss. It is imperative to ensure effective symptom management during the dying process to aid a family's grief. **Table 2** highlights some of the changes that one can experience during the dying process as described through the human senses. It is important to proactively educate parents on expected symptoms and planned interventions to help parents become aware of their child's symptoms, thus leading to a better understanding and ability to manage expectations.[16] Proactively reviewing these experiences also normalizes them, which can grant caregivers peace that these symptoms are expected, normal, and can be treated.

Table 2
Sensory experience at the end of life

See	Skin changes, including color (pallor, cyanosis), mottling especially of distal body parts, including hands, feet, elbows, and knees Decreased activity, more time spent sleeping, may appear withdrawn Decreased responsiveness, difficulty awakening, may become unresponsive Changes in behavior, including agitation and confusion
Hear	Variable respiratory patterns including shallow, deep, labored, and apnea Secretions, "death rattle," loss of control of oropharyngeal muscles
Feel	Touch: temperature changes; both warm (fevers) and progressive coolness Changes in heart beat; both rapid and slow with weakening of pulses peripherally Emotions: anxiety, anger, guilt, confusion, fear, relief, incompetency, ambivalence, uncertainty, and loneliness
Smell	Urine and stool from bladder and bowel incontinence as pelvic muscles relax Changes in breath odor (eg, ketotic)
Taste	Skin and lips may taste salty with dehydration

Courtesy of J. Hirsh, MD, Columbus, OH.

Honoring the Caregiver's Role in Pediatric End-of-Life Care

Case: You have been consulted by the neonatal intensive care unit (NICU) due to conflict between a father and the staff. His daughter, Sophia, born 2 weeks ago, has extensive anoxic brain injury and an examination very worrisome for global neurologic injury. The NICU has already met with the parents and relayed her grave neurologic prognosis. This meeting ended abruptly when dad voiced anger that he and his wife have been robbed of the ability to be parents at the bedside throughout the hospitalization. He cited several examples in which he or his wife felt pushed aside so that nursing staff could perform cares. You have been asked to assist in conflict resolution.

Concomitant with empowering caregivers with this knowledge is the need to adopt a shared process model that incorporates both medical and parental priorities to best preserve the parents' role and their relationship with their child.[17] The impending death of a child threatens the previously established definition of what it means to be a parent.[18,19] Moreover, as health care providers step in to manage end-of-life symptoms, parents can be inadvertently left feeling marginalized or inept in their capacity to comfort their child. Research shows that parents wish to be recognized for their continued responsibility and contribution to their child's care, especially in the last moments.[20] Including parents in shared decision making allows them to feel empowered before, during, and even after their child dies. Near the end of life, not only is it important to provide this anticipatory guidance, but also to provide privacy, dignity, and a peaceful family-centered environment.[21]

Such family-centered care includes highlighting to parents their ability to provide non-pharmacological comfort interventions during end-of-life care. At times, one does not need to do or say anything, simply being present provides a sense of comfort. This includes educating parents on the following:

- Plan for visitors during times when the child is most alert
- Familiar voices provide comfort and reassurance:
  - Talk, read, and sing to the child
  - Play the child's favorite song, share favorite memories
  - Remember that laughter and sadness can coincide

- Refocus feeding as a pleasure and not a nutritional goal by letting the child guide choices and give permission to not eat or drink if unpleasant
- For older children, as bowel and bladder changes occur, ensure privacy and be sure that the child is kept dry and comfortable
- When noisy breathing occurs
  - Remember that this is a natural part of the dying process and there is no indication that it represents pain or suffering
  - Consider gently turning the child on his or her side and raising the head of bed, which can help decrease this sound
- Provide comforting blankets to make it feel like home wherever they are
- Offer gentle touch or even massage; this offers great love and support
- If the child develops confusion,
  - Remind the child that you will keep him or her safe
  - Surround the child with familiar objects and people to assist in reorientation if possible
- For older children, listen carefully; there may be meaningful messages in symbolic language (eg, "I want to go home") and having the courage to ask, "tell me more"
- Follow your heart when saying goodbye, as there is no single right way to do this

SUMMARY

With the ever-changing advances in pediatric health care, pediatric death is becoming an ever-growing rarity. Mental health care providers can provide a crucial role in ensuring support to family members who face this loss. This is best achieved by facilitating re-goaling in those caregivers capable of such achievements followed by anticipatory guidance that focuses on symptom education, prognostication grounded in symptoms, and augmenting the role of the caregiver in providing nonpharmacological interventions to mitigate these symptoms. Such actions can better ensure that caregivers are supported before, during, and after the devastation that is the loss of a child.

REFERENCES

1. Wilson DC. The ultimate loss: the dying child. Loss, Grief & Care 1988;2(3–4): 125–30.
2. Brown E, Dominica F. Around the time of death: culture, religion, and ritual. In: Goldman A, Hain R, Liben S, editors. Oxford textbook of palliative care for children. 2nd edition. New York: Oxford University Press Inc; 2012. p. 142–54.
3. Kars MC, Grypdonck MH, Beishuizen A, et al. Factors influencing parental readiness to let their child with cancer die. Pediatr Blood Cancer 2010;54(7):1000–8.
4. Feudtner C, Walter JK, Faerber JA, et al. Good-parent beliefs of parents of seriously ill children. JAMA Pediatr 2015;169(1):39–47.
5. Aging with dignity © 2018. Available at: https://www.agingwithdignity.org. Accessed May 9, 2018.
6. Coda alliance © 2016. Available at: https://codaalliance.org/go-wish/. Accessed May 9, 2018.
7. Christakis NA, Lamont EB. Extent and determinants of error in doctors' prognoses in terminally ill patients: prospective cohort study. BMJ 2000;320:469–72.
8. Brook L, Hain R. Predicting death in children. Arch Dis Child 2008;93(12): 1067–70.
9. Hendricks-Ferguson V. Physical symptoms of children receiving pediatric hospice care at home during the last week of life. Oncol Nurs Forum 2008;35(6): E108–15.

10. Kars MC, Grypdonck MH, van Delden JJ. Being a parent of a child with cancer throughout the end-of-life course. Oncol Nurs Forum 2011;38(4):E260–71.
11. Wolfe J, Grier HE, Klar N, et al. Symptoms and suffering at the end of life in children with cancer. N Engl J Med 2000;342(5):326–33.
12. Hechler T, Blankenburg M, Friedrichsdorf SJ, et al. Parents' perspective on symptoms, quality of life, characteristics of death and end-of-life decisions for children dying from cancer. Klin Padiatr 2008;220(3):166–74.
13. Pritchard M, Burghen E, Srivastava DK, et al. Cancer-related symptoms most concerning to parents during the last week and last day of their child's life. Pediatrics 2008;121(5):e1301–9.
14. Drake R, Frost J, Collins JJ. The symptoms of dying children. J Pain Symptom Manage 2003;26(1):594–603.
15. Pritchard M, Burghen EA, Gattuso JS, et al. Factors that distinguish symptoms of most concern to parents from other symptoms of dying children. J Pain Symptom Manage 2010;39(4):627–36.
16. Hinds PS, Oakes LL, Hicks J, et al. End-of-life care for children and adolescents. Semin Oncol Nurs 2005;21(1):53–62.
17. Lamiani G, Giannini A, Fossati I, et al. Parental experience of end-of life care in the pediatric intensive care unit. Minerva Anestesiol 2013;79(12):1334–43.
18. Miles M, Carter M, Riddle L, et al. The pediatric intensive care unit as a source of stress for parents. Matern Child Health J 1989;18:199–206.
19. Meert KL, Thurston CS, Ashok AP. End-of-life decision-making and satisfaction with care: parental perspectives. Pediatr Crit Care Med 2000;1:179–85.
20. Longden JV. Parental perceptions of end-of-life care on paediatric intensive care units: a literature review. Nurs Crit Care 2011;16(3):131–9.
21. Davies D. Care in the final hours and days. In: Goldman A, Hain R, Liben S, editors. Oxford textbook of palliative care for children. 2nd edition. New York: Oxford University Press Inc.; 2012. p. 368–74.

Ethical Issues Around Pediatric Death

Navigating Consent, Assent, and Disagreement Regarding Life-Sustaining Medical Treatment

Silvana Barone, MD[a], Yoram Unguru, MD, MS, MA[b,c],*

KEYWORDS

- Consent • Assent • Death • Life-sustaining medical treatment • Adolescents
- Decision-making

KEY POINTS

- The principle of pediatric assent recognizes the need to recognize and respect the wishes of children as they develop cognitively and mature.
- Health care providers should provide developmentally appropriate disclosures about illness and solicit the child's willingness and preferences regarding treatment to a level that is commensurate with their decision-making capacity.
- Adolescents displaying psychosocial maturity should be given a larger role in decision-making, including decisions regarding their end-of-life care.
- When prognosis is poor and disagreement arises regarding the use of experimental therapy or life-sustaining medical treatment, every effort must be made to explore goals and values and reach a consensus on the therapeutic plan.

INTRODUCTION

In modern society, we expect parents to outlive their children. Childhood death is a difficult reality, in part, because it defies the expected order of life events, challenging basic existential assumptions and threatening parental roles of protecting offspring.[1,2] The death of a child is one of the most painful events a family can experience and is associated with complicated and traumatic grief reactions.[3,4] In the United States,

---

[a] Division of General Pediatrics and Adolescent Medicine, The Johns Hopkins Hospital, Johns Hopkins University Berman Institute of Bioethics, 200 North Wolfe Street, Baltimore, MD 21287, USA; [b] Division of Pediatric Hematology/Oncology, The Herman and Walter Samuelson Children's Hospital at Sinai, 2401 West Belvedere Avenue, Baltimore, MD 21215, USA; [c] Johns Hopkins University Berman Institute of Bioethics, 1809 Ashland Avenue, Baltimore, MD 21205, USA
* Corresponding author. Division of Pediatric Hematology/Oncology, The Herman & Walter Samuelson Children's Hospital at Sinai, 2401 West Belvedere Avenue, Baltimore, MD 21215.
E-mail address: yunguru@lifebridgehealth.org

Child Adolesc Psychiatric Clin N Am 27 (2018) 539–550
https://doi.org/10.1016/j.chc.2018.05.009
1056-4993/18/© 2018 Elsevier Inc. All rights reserved.

childpsych.theclinics.com

between 40,000 and 50,000 children die every year from trauma, lethal congenital conditions, extreme prematurity, heritable disorders, or acquired illness.[5] Of these, more than 1500 are adolescents who die of the effects of chronic illness, including malignant neoplasms, heart disease and congenital malformations, and chromosomal anomalies.[5]

Health care providers (HCPs) caring for children with life-limiting illness face many challenges, including, but not limited to, management of distressing symptoms, difficult conversations about prognosis and goals of care, facilitating longitudinal decision-making in the face of prognostic uncertainty, and navigating conflict with family members and other HCPs.[6–9] For example, conflict in pediatric end of life can occur if parents ask HCPs not to disclose a poor prognosis to their child, even when cure is exceedingly unlikely. These requests can lead to moral distress for HCPs who must navigate tensions between coexisting principles of avoiding harm and enabling autonomy, while striving to uphold their professional integrity for truth telling.[2,10] Furthermore, disagreement about the goals of medical care can be an important source of conflict; family members may disagree with medical recommendations because of different perceptions and expectations about the child's quality of life, different interpretations of the prognosis, or religious and culturally based beliefs that influence their sense of what is best.[11] Disagreement within the health care team about the direction of care may also occur, leading to fragmented caregiving and the communication of inconsistent or conflicting information to families.[12] For children with life-limiting illness, questions surrounding the use of experimental therapies or life-sustaining medical treatment (LSMT) often arise and can be a significant source of conflict and distress for both the health care team and the child-family dyad. How are such decisions made for these seriously ill children? Do, and should, children have a say in their care when their choices represent, quite literally, life and death decisions? If the answer to this question is yes, what would this look like in practice and, importantly, should limitations on a child's decision-making exist? The following sections explore issues related to pediatric decision-making in cases of incurable disease and provide some guidance for HCPs navigating these often emotionally charged and ethically challenging clinical situations.

Decision-Making for Minors with Life-Limiting Illness: Concepts of Consent, Assent, and Emerging Capacity

The pediatric model of patient- and family centered care recognizes that patients and their families are integral partners with the health care team and that the child and family's perspectives are essential components of high-quality clinical decision-making.[13] With a few exceptions,[14] parents are granted authority to make medical decisions on behalf of minor children, including adolescents. Parents are generally afforded a great deal of discretion in terms of the choices they make, so long as their choices do not place the child at risk of serious harm as compared with the alternatives.[15,16]

For children with chronic life-limiting illness, medical decision-making is not a discrete event but a process whereby families assimilate new information and make decisions over time as the child's clinical condition evolves and, often, deteriorates. Such decisions can include whether to proceed with surgeries for a feeding tube and tracheostomy for progressive dysphagia and respiratory failure or whether to pursue further courses of aggressive chemotherapy for cancer after initial treatments have failed. Given the potential consequences of severe disability and/or death of the child, the process whereby these decisions are made can be fraught with challenges and conflict for both families and HCPs.

PEDIATRIC CONSENT AND ASSENT

By definition, children constitute a vulnerable population, relating directly to their limited decision-making capacity (ie, the ability to make reasonable decisions).[17] Children and adolescents with incurable conditions have extra sources of vulnerability; they may experience significant emotional and psychological distress related to their prognosis.[18,19] Furthermore, older children and adolescents with chronic illness often depend on parents or HCPs for many aspects of daily living (bathing, feeding, ambulating) at a time when otherwise healthy children are exploring and benefiting from their burgeoning independence.[20] As the appropriate surrogate decision-makers for minors, only parents (or legal guardians) can legally provide permission (consent) to treatment and procedures for their child. Informed consent incorporates the following 3 duties:

1. Disclosure of information to patients and their surrogates
2. Assessment of patient and surrogate understanding of the information and their capacity for medical decision-making
3. Obtaining informed consent before treatments and interventions[21]

The current notion of informed consent in medical practice finds it support in ethical theory in the concept of autonomy, which is understood as the right of an autonomous agent to make decisions as guided by his or her own reason.[22] The goals of the informed consent process, which include protecting and promoting health-related interests and incorporating the patients and/or families in health care decision-making, apply to both the pediatric and adult population and are grounded in the same ethical principles of beneficence, justice, and respect for autonomy.

The principle of pediatric *assent* recognizes that children (especially adolescents) are capable of participating in decision-making related to their care and provides a process by which to meet these goals for children and adolescents who cannot legally provide informed consent. In the United States, 18 years of age is considered the age of maturity and the legal age at which adolescents are considered competent to make their own decisions. However, child health and legal experts acknowledge there is no specific cutoff age at which a child or adolescent suddenly acquires full decision-making capacity. Rather, the assent requirement calls for the need to recognize and respect the wishes of children as they develop cognitively and mature.[17] A developmental approach to assent anticipates different levels of understanding from children as they age.[23] Age alone, however, fails to adequately determine a child's ability to make meaningful decisions. Knowledge, health status, anxiety, experience with decision-making, and each child's unique cultural, familial, religious background, and values all play a role in children's understanding of their situation and impact their ability to make decisions.[17] Children living with serious illness often experience a loss of control over their bodies, their social lives, and their ability to make choices for themselves.[20] Yet, at the same time, by virtue of their lived experience, these children often possess a degree of decision-making capacity. Thus, the process of seeking assent is one way for HCPs to empower children to the extent of their capacity.[17] When seeking assent, HCPs should help the patient achieve a developmentally appropriate awareness of his or her condition and perform a clinical assessment of the patient's understanding of the situation before they can solicit an expression of the patient's willingness to accept the proposed care. This process must also include an assessment of factors that may influence the patient's response, including inappropriate pressure to accept testing or therapy.[21]

EMERGING CAPACITY IN CHILDREN AND ADOLESCENTS

Empirical studies of cognitive development in children suggest that many minors reach the formal operational stage of cognitive development that allows abstract thinking and the ability to handle complex tasks by midadolescence.[24,25] The most widely cited study on adolescents' capacity for rational decision-making was published nearly 40 years ago and concluded that by the 14 years of age, adolescents are as able as adults to make rational and reasonable health care decisions.[24] Furthermore, some have suggested that experience with chronic illness can enhance the ability of children and adolescents to develop capacity to make health care decisions.[26,27] However, an adolescent's ability for adultlike decision-making does not guarantee such decisions. Moreover, whether an adolescent is capable of adultlike decision-making does not necessarily determine whether these decisions should be respected. More recently, advanced imaging techniques, such as functional MRI, and clinical neuropsychological evaluation have provided additional insight into decision-making capacity and processes. Diekema[15] argues that although adolescents may be capable of adultlike decision-making, they do not perform at a level commensurate with their cognitive abilities. They are more affected by the influence of peers, less future oriented, more impulsive, and differ in their assessment of risks and rewards as compared with adults. Insofar as decision-making capacity, although adolescents may possess the right equipment to allow for such capacity, they have yet to fully master its implementation. Psychologists distinguish between cold and hot cognition. Cold cognitive abilities are those used in calm situations with little to no peer influence and time to deliberate and reason logically with facts. Studies of cold cognition have shown that the skills necessary to make informed decisions are firmly in place by 16 years of age.[28] By that age, adolescents can gather and process information, weigh pros and cons, reason logically with facts, and take time before making a decision.[29] This finding suggests that under ideal conditions, adolescents are often as able as their adult counterparts to make health care–related decisions; however, ideal conditions are rare. Hot cognitive abilities are those used to make decisions in situations of emotional arousal or conflict, when there is peer influence and/or time pressure. In these situations, the most critical skill is self-regulation, which enables an individual to control emotions, withstand pressures from others, and check impulses.[29] Hot and cold cognition are subserved by different neuronal circuits and have different developmental courses.[30] From a neurobiological standpoint, in emotionally charged situations and decisions made under stressful conditions (eg, life-limiting illness), adolescents may rely on their more mature limbic systems than the less mature prefrontal control system.[15,31] The prefrontal cortex is the region of the brain responsible for high-level reasoning, executive function, weighing consequences, planning, organization, and emotional regulation. Rational decision-making is the last faculty to mature. In fact, brain development is not finalized well into the 20s.[32]

There exist circumstances in which a minor may legally make decisions regarding his or her own health care. Throughout the United States, medically emancipated minor acts permit minors to make medical decisions for specific conditions without parental involvement. These conditions include sexually transmitted infections, substance abuse, pregnancy, and psychiatric services. Medically emancipated minor acts largely exist because of public health concerns and did not result from respect for adolescents' evolving capacity. Mature minor status affords some adolescents the authority to make medical decisions beyond the aforementioned conditions. Minor treatment statutes in some states, known as the mature minor doctrine, allow minors with *adequate decisional capacity and understanding* of their medical condition the right to consent to treatment without parental permission.[33] This doctrine applies to nonemancipated minors who understand the risks and benefits of treatment and applies only to specific medical decisions. Under this doctrine, the age, overall maturity, cognitive abilities, and social situation of the minor are considered in a judicial determination, finding that an otherwise legally incompetent minor is sufficiently mature to make a legally binding decision and provide his or her own consent for medical care.[14] Mature minor standards vary by state.[33] Increasingly, professional medical organizations support mature minor doctrine, allowing physicians to treat minors without parental permission (consent) even in states that lack specific mature minor statutes.[14,34,35] Age plays a role in mature minor doctrine, with 16 years of age being the common cutoff; but in some states minors as young as 14 years are granted the right to consent to any medical treatment without parental permission (consent). Lastly, emancipated minors are a select group of adolescents deemed by the legal system to meet specific criteria allowing them to consent to their own care. Qualifications to be considered emancipated include minors who are married, active military, and living on their own and managing their own finances.

Even when not fully autonomous, older children and adolescents can be considered to fall somewhere on a spectrum of emerging capacity in decision-making. A child's decision is deemed valid so long as they choose freely (voluntarily), their choice is reasonable and rationale, and they understand information relevant to their choice.[36] Assent in this context can be defined as the inclusion of a minor child, to the extent possible, in receiving information and making decisions regarding his or her health care, even when the child is not yet legally able to provide true informed consent.[37] No universal standard defines decision-making capacity. A child's ability to make a substantive decision depends on the type of decision and the risks and benefits involved. What is clear is that children develop decisional capacity in stages, and children of differing ages have differing abilities. Capacity is linked both to developing cognition and to prior life experiences.[17] When considering whether to respect an adolescent's decision, one approach is the threshold level of capacity whereby high-risk decisions require a higher threshold, low-risk decisions require a lower threshold, and the remaining decisions are somewhere in between. Ultimately, decision-making capacity is not an all or none phenomenon. When determining a minor's ability to make a meaningful decision, the question is whether a *given* child possesses the capacity for a *particular* decision. Ethically, a child may possess the skills to participate in some health care–related decision-making while lacking the skills for other decisions. Standards of practice promoted by the National Hospice and Palliative Care Organization call for physicians to seek assent and take into consideration dissent of older children and adolescents who demonstrate some health care decision-making capacity, "while ensuring the child's best interests remain at the core of decisions."[38]

What Happens When Minors and Their Parents Disagree?

Marjorie is a 16-year-old girl with an aggressive form of leukemia for which she has undergone 2 cycles of chemotherapy. Her cancer and its treatment have left her with distressing symptoms, including neuropathic pain, mouth sores, and extreme fatigue. Marjorie is a good student and loves to dance. Because of her illness, she has had to leave school and the dance team. She lives with her parents and 14-year-old sister. Today, she and her parents met with the oncologist who compassionately explained that the cancer has relapsed and that further aggressive chemotherapy is unlikely to lead to cure. Marjorie has previously met with members of the palliative care team including the child life specialist and has had a chance to discuss her goals and wishes with them as well as her parents. Marjorie and her parents agree that pursuing chemotherapy does not fit with Marjorie's previously expressed wishes of going to the beach one last time with her family and spending her remaining time at home with family rather than full of tubes in the pediatric intensive care unit. Following the meeting with the oncologist, Marjorie and her mother met with the palliative care team again to discuss the best way to honor her wishes moving forward, and a referral to hospice care is made. Given that Marjorie already has a therapeutic relationship with members of the palliative care team, meeting with them again does not feel new and scary. Marjorie returned home with a plan for management of pain and dyspnea. She was able to go to the beach with her family for 2 days. Over the following weeks, she made a video for her sister and prepared a box of dance memorabilia to share with the dance team. As she began to feel weaker, the hospice nurse came to the house more often to help with symptom relief. Marjorie died peacefully at home surrounded by loved ones.

This scenario likely represents the best possible outcome in a tragic situation when death is inevitable. Marjorie, her parents, and her health care team agreed on a care plan that prioritized Marjorie's comfort and desire to spend her last few weeks at the beach and at home with loved ones rather than in the hospital.

What happens when a minor and his or her parents do not agree on the best course of action? Children and adolescents may refuse further LSMT, whereas parents ask for continued aggressive therapy or experimental treatments. The authors limit their discussion to disagreement and conflicts that arise in the specific case of life-limiting, incurable illness whereby death is expected to result regardless of medical interventions (acknowledging that there can be a great deal of uncertainty with regard to the timeline for clinical deterioration and death). A minor and/or his or her parents' refusal of potentially life-saving therapy (eg, chemotherapy for highly curable form of cancer) remains contentious, as evidenced by several high-profile US court cases. A 2007 Virginia court case (*Virginia v Cherrix*) centered around 15-year-old Starchild Abraham Cherrix's refusal to undergo further chemotherapy for Hodgkin lymphoma, a highly treatable and curable form of cancer. His parents supported his choice and were subsequently accused by the state of medical neglect of their child. The parties reached a compromise in a consent decree, in which Cherrix would receive treatment from a board-certified specialist of his choice for alternative therapies.[39] The case resulted in the enactment of Abraham's Law, which increased the rights of minor patients aged 14 to 17 years in Virginia to refuse medical treatment. According to Abraham's Law, for children with a life-threatening illness at least 14 years old, parents cannot be charged with medical neglect for refusing medically recommended treatment if

1. The decision is made jointly by the child and parents.
2. The child is sufficiently mature to have an informed opinion on the treatment.
3. Other treatments have been considered.
4. They believe in good faith that their choice is in the child's best interest.[40]

Courts have sided with adolescents who refuse lifesaving therapies in the case of Billy Best (a 16 year old with Hodgkin lymphoma) and Dennis Lindberg (a 14 year old with acute lymphoblastic leukemia). Best refused additional therapy for personal reasons, whereas Lindberg was a practicing Jehovah's Witness who refused blood transfusions for religious reasons. Further complicating the situation was the fact that Lindberg's aunt, who was his legal guardian, supported his decision, whereas his biological parents did not. Examples of courts overturning patient/parental refusal of lifesaving chemotherapy include the cases of Daniel Hauser (a 12 year old with Hodgkin lymphoma), Jeremy Fraser (a 7 year old with non-Hodgkin lymphoma), and Cassandra Callender (a 16 year old with Hodgkin lymphoma).

With the exception of the Callender case, there seems to be a clear distinction between the courts' willingness to support children and parents who refuse lifesaving chemotherapy for cancer when the child is young and when the child is older (>14 years of age). Although the issue of refusal of efficacious treatment of minors with life-limiting illness remains controversial, the trend among the courts and state legislatures is toward being increasingly more tolerant of permitting refusal, especially when the minor and parents are in agreement. From the clinician's perspective, it is reasonable to contend that in clinical situations when the benefits of treatment clearly outweigh the risks and burdens (eg, starting fluids and intravenous antibiotics for suspected sepsis), adolescents should not be allowed to refuse life-saving treatment, even when parents agree.[15,34,41] Similarly, parental refusals of care for their minor child should not be honored in such situations. Although pediatric assent is ethically important, ultimately, parental permission may trump assent and is legally binding. However, in clinical scenarios where prognosis is poor and potential medical interventions are associated with a heavy patient burden, it seems reasonable to provide sufficient considerations to the adolescent's opportunity to provide assent or refusal.[21]

STANDARDS FOR PEDIATRIC DECISION-MAKING

Historically, medical decision-making for minors has centered on the best-interest standard (BIS), which directs the surrogate to maximize benefits and minimize harms to the minor.[42] Conflicts surrounding end-of-life decision-making centered on forgoing or discontinuing LSMT often stem from disagreement over different ideas about what constitutes the patients' best interest. Regardless of associated burdens, some parents might think that maintaining life is the only worthwhile goal and, therefore, all efforts should be directed toward sustaining and/or prolonging the life of their child. Adolescents might place more emphasis on functional abilities and quality of life and want to have a say in where and how they spend their final days and weeks. Although the BIS has become the moral foundation of clinical pediatric ethics, it is also a topic of much debate among pediatric bioethicists. In fact, some argue that it is an impossible standard to uphold.[16,43,44] Part of the problem relates to consent. Consent is literally defined as "to feel or to sense,"[45] and expresses something for one's self. In consenting, a person does so based on their own personal beliefs or values. Therefore, critics of the BIS state that it is individualistic, making parents' interests paramount, placing burdens on the interests of others.[44] Importantly, no person can consent for another person, rather they may give their permission. Therefore, when discussing a parent's decision for their child, permission is the accepted term.

Rather than rely on the BIS, which is highly subjective, Rhodes and Holzman[44] propose that parents should be held to a not unreasonable standard, whereby parents' decisions would be respected unless they were deemed unreasonable. Reasonable parents acting in good faith may choose differently from other parents facing similar situations, and yet both sets of parents might be judged as acting in their child's best interest.[37] This standard might prove more helpful in situations when the best interest of patients is the source of disagreement but does not resolve the enduring controversy about informed refusal of LSMT by adolescents.[41,46,47]

COLLABORATIVE COMMUNICATION IN END-OF-LIFE CARE

The health care team is primarily responsible for determining whether an adolescent's refusal represents a reasonable choice. As alluded to, due to neurobiological developments, adolescents may not make decisions commensurate with their decision-making capacity. However, exceptions can be made for adolescents who can demonstrate not simply the ability to understand and reason, but who also possess a high level of psychosocial maturity. Components of psychosocial maturity that develop during adolescence include:

1. The ability to control impulses including aggressive impulses;
2. The ability to consider other points of view, including those that take into account longer term consequences or that take the vantage point of others; and
3. The ability to take personal responsibility for one's behavior and resist the coercive influences of others.[48]

A component of evaluating psychosocial maturity would require HCPs to perform an assessment of the adolescent's ability to project meaningfully into the future, express a relatively settled set of values and beliefs, and demonstrate that their decision is driven more by long-term interests than short-term concerns. Even when HCPs can make this determination, the challenge of reconciling among family members remains. Rarely, HCPs might question whether parents are truly acting in their child's best interest as may occur when parental decisions have the potential for inflicting an unacceptable amount of harm on their child. For the child receiving palliative care, this occurs when parents request specific treatment (eg, experimental therapies with significant risks and doubtful benefits) or refuse others (eg, adequate analgesia at the end-of-life).[37] In these situations, HCPs must recognize that for some parents of seriously ill children, making the medical decisions and advocating for their child until the very end may be necessary for them to feel they are "good parents."[49] The decision to "leave no stone unturned" may be critical to their definition of good parenting.[10] The process of end-of-life decision-making must be respectful of parents' needs and the fact that once the child has died, the parents are left to grapple with any decisional regret they may have.

When parents continue to speak in hopeful terms about their child's prognosis after HCPs have communicated otherwise, HCPs sometimes lament that *parents just don't get it*. Similarly, HCPs may be confused when children who are thought to understand their prognosis speak in front of their parents about what college they will attend or what job they will have when they grow up. These behaviors can be partly explained by the concept of mutual pretense, which argues that children are extensions of larger social networks and that illness can influence a child to try to maintain their role, and the role of other family members, as they existed *before* becoming sick.[50] Accordingly, illness can cause a child to conceal their true desires and understanding in an effort to preserve the status quo. In mutual pretense, all parties in the therapeutic relationship know what is going to happen, but they fail to discuss this knowledge with one another. By engaging in mutual pretense, children prevent the child-parent and patient-doctor relationship from falling apart. This mutual pretense calls into question whether open and honest discussions between children, parents, and physicians about substantive issues like relapse/refractory disease can ever occur. At the very least, knowledge of mutual pretense by HCPs may mitigate misunderstandings between HCPs and family members, thus, improving communication and minimizing conflict during difficult discussions. Related, when parents and children disagree about the best course of action, it is crucial to explore with parents their reasons for

---

Box 1
Strategies for minimizing conflict and improving care for children with life-limiting illness

- Set clear expectations for open and honest communication early in the therapeutic relationship; inform parents you will always be honest with their child.

- Ascertain the type, as well as how much, information children and adolescents want to receive about their condition and prognosis; deliver the information using developmentally appropriate language tailored to the individual child's abilities or developmental level.

- Whenever appropriate, solicit the child's assent.

- Following initial diagnosis of a life-limiting condition, involve a pediatric palliative care team early. When cure is unlikely or impossible, engage in deliberative communication regarding the patient and family's values and goals of care.

- Engage adolescents in discussions on legacy making and preferences for end-of-life care (advance care planning); include parents in these discussions when possible.

- Seek help from consultants in palliative care and/or ethics teams when disagreement exists about the role of experimental therapy and/or LSMT.

---

pursuing LSMT or experimental therapies and to allow the adolescent the opportunity to articulate why he or she wishes to forego such therapies. Often, drawing from medical expertise and the adolescent's previously articulated goals, the HCP can thoughtfully describe how pursuing LSMT would not be in line with these goals. Furthermore, although HCPs must endeavor to be respectful and explore the family's values and cultural/religious practices, they are under no obligation to provide care they feel is unethical or harmful (eg, failing to provide adequate analgesia).[2]

The child's decision not to pursue LSMT can certainly be considered reasonable when there is a high degree of probability that treatment is clearly ineffective or harmful or that life will be severely shortened regardless of treatment. It is, therefore, ethically permissible and even advisable for the health care team to make a medical recommendation to the family against pursuing LSMT and shift the focus to greater palliative and comfort care. Parents should not think that the health care team is ganging up on them or giving up on their child but rather that HCPs are thoughtfully and respectfully considering the child's wishes and goals for comfort in the context of the family unit and the medical information at their disposal. This understanding requires that both HCPs and families commit time and effort for deliberative communication that explores individual and shared values and allows for evolving moral opinions and needs.[10] In these difficult situations, support from palliative care consultants, social workers, child life specialists, and/or psychologists is invaluable. Additionally, an ethics consultation team can also provide insight on the ethical permissibility of different courses of action. Legal recourse should be a last resort, pursued only if all other options have been exhausted and disagreement remains. Strategies for facilitating conciliatory communication about end-of life decision-making can be found in **Box 1**.

SUMMARY

Caring for children with a life-limiting illness can be a challenging, albeit rewarding, task for clinicians. All children and adolescents, regardless of physical or mental disability, have a right to medical treatment that respects their dignity and intrinsic value as persons. HCPs should provide developmentally appropriate disclosure about illness and solicit the child's willingness and preferences regarding treatment to a level that is commensurate with their decision-making capacity. Adolescents displaying psychosocial maturity should be given a larger role in decision-making, including decisions regarding their end-of-life care. When disagreement between parents and children around the use of noncurative therapy or LSMT exists, HCPs should use all resources at their disposal with the goal of achieving consensus within the family.

REFERENCES

1. Wheeler I. Parental bereavement: the crisis of meaning. Death Stud 2001;25(1): 51–66.
2. Rosenberg AR, Starks H, Unguru Y, et al. Truth telling in the setting of cultural differences and incurable pediatric illness: a review. JAMA Pediatr 2017;171(11): 1113–9.
3. Prigerson HG, Shear MK, Jacobs SC, et al. Consensus criteria for traumatic grief: a preliminary empirical test. Br J Psychiatry 1999;174:67–73.
4. Rogers CH, Floyd FJ, Seltzer MM, et al. Long-term effects of the death of a dhild on parents' adjustment in midlife. J Fam Psychol 2008;22(2):203–11.
5. Murphy SL, Mathews TJ, Martin JA, et al. Annual summary of vital statistics: 2013-2014. Pediatrics 2017;139(6) [pii:e20163239].
6. Doorenbos A, Lindhorst T, Starks H, et al. Palliative care in the pediatric ICU: challenges and opportunities for family-centered practice. J Soc Work End Life Palliat Care 2012;8(4):297–315.
7. Hilden JM, Himelstein BP, Freyer DR, et al. End-of-life care: special issues in pediatric oncology. In: Institute of Medicine (US) and National Research Council (US) National Cancer Policy Board, Foley KM, Gelband H, editors. Improving palliative care for cancer. Washington, DC: National Academies Press; 2001. p. 6. Available at: https://www.ncbi.nlm.nih.gov/books/NBK223531/. Accessed Febuary 27, 2018.
8. Lipstein EA, Britto MT. The evolution of pediatric chronic disease treatment decisions: a qualitative, longitudinal view of parents' decision-making process. Med Decis Making 2015;35(6):703–13.
9. Marcus KL, Henderson CM, Boss RD. Chronic critical illness in infants and children: a speculative synthesis on adapting ICU care to meet the needs of long-stay patients. Pediatr Crit Care Med 2016;17(8):743–52.
10. Rosenberg AR, Wolfe J, Wiener L, et al. Ethics, emotions, and the skills of talking about progressing disease with terminally ill adolescents: a review. JAMA Pediatr 2016;170(12):1216–23.
11. Weise KL, Okun AL, Carter BS, et al. Guidance on forgoing life-sustaining medical treatment. Pediatrics 2017;140(3) [pii:e20171905].
12. Nelson JE. Identifying and overcoming the barriers to high-quality palliative care in the intensive care unit. Crit Care Med 2006;34(11 Suppl):S324–31.
13. Committee On Hospital Care and Institute For Patient- and Family-Centered Care. Patient- and family-centered care and the pediatrician's role. Pediatrics 2012; 129(2):394–404.
14. Katz AL, Webb SA, Committee on Bioethics. Informed consent in decision-making in pediatric practice. Pediatrics 2016;138(2) [pii:e20161485].
15. Diekema DS. Adolescent refusal of lifesaving treatment: are we asking the right questions? Adolesc Med State Art Rev 2011;22(2):213–28, viii.
16. Diekema DS. Parental refusals of medical treatment: the harm principle as threshold for state intervention. Theor Med Bioeth 2004;25(4):243–64.

17. Unguru Y. Making sense of adolescent decision-making: challenge and reality. Adolesc Med State Art Rev 2011;22(2):195–206, vii-viii.
18. Collins JJ, Devine TD, Dick GS, et al. The measurement of symptoms in young children with cancer: the validation of the Memorial Symptom Assessment Scale in children aged 7-12. J Pain Symptom Manage 2002;23(1):10–6.
19. Compas BE, Jaser SS, Dunn MJ, et al. Coping with chronic illness in childhood and adolescence. Annu Rev Clin Pyschol 2012;8:455–80.
20. Yeo M, Sawyer S. Chronic illness and disability. BMJ 2005;330(7493):721–3.
21. Committee on Bioethics. Informed consent in decision-making in pediatric practice. Pediatrics 2016;138(2) [pii:e20161484].
22. Beauchamp TL, Children JF. Principles of biomedical ethics. 5th edition. New York: Oxford University Press; 2001.
23. Miller VA, Nelson RM. A developmental approach to child assent for nontherapeutic research. J Pediatr 2006;149(1 Suppl):S25–30.
24. Weithorn LA, Campbell SB. The competency of children and adolescents to make informed treatment decisions. Child Dev 1982;53(6):1589–98.
25. McCabe MA. Involving children and adolescents in medical decision making: developmental and clinical considerations. J Pediatr Psychol 1996;21(4):505–16.
26. Alderson P. Competent children? Minors' consent to health care treatment and research. Soc Sci Med 2007;65(11):2272–83.
27. Alderson P, Sutcliffe K, Curtis K. Children's competence to consent to medical treatment. Hastings Cent Rep 2006;36(6):25–34.
28. Steinberg L, Cauffman E, Woolard J, et al. Are adolescents less mature than adults?: minors' access to abortion, the juvenile death penalty, and the alleged APA "flip-flop". Am Psychol 2009;64(7):583–94.
29. Steinberg L. Why we should lower the voting age to 16. The New York Times 2018. Available at: https://www.nytimes.com/2018/03/02/opinion/sunday/voting-age-school-shootings.html. Accessed March 4, 2018.
30. Steinberg L. Cognitive and affective development in adolescence. Trends Cogn Sci 2005;9(2):69–74.
31. Casey B, Jones RM, Somerville LH. Braking and accelerating of the adolescent brain. J Res Adolesc 2011;21(1):21–33.
32. Steinberg L. Does recent research on adolescent brain development inform the mature minor doctrine? J Med Philos 2013;38(3):256–67.
33. Coleman DL, Rosoff PM. The legal authority of mature minors to consent to general medical treatment. Pediatrics 2013;131(4):786–93.
34. Harrison C. Treatment decisions regarding infants, children and adolescents. J Paediatr Child Health 2004;9(2):99–114.
35. AMA code of medical ethics' opinion on adolescent care. Virtual Mentor 2014; 16(11):901–2.
36. Unguru Y. American Academy of Pediatrics bioethics resident curriculum: case-based teaching guides. Session 3: informed consent and assent in clinical pediatrics. 2017. Available at: https://www.aap.org/en-us/Documents/Bioethics-InformedConsent.pdf. Accessed March 4, 2018.
37. Rapoport A, Morrison W. No child is an island: ethical considerations in end-of-life care for children and their families. Curr Opin Support Palliat Care 2016;10(3): 196–200.
38. National Hospice and Palliative Care Orgnization. Standards of practice for pediatric palliative care and hospice. 2009. Available at: https://www.nhpco.org/sites/default/files/public/quality/Ped_Pall_Care%20_Standard.pdf.pdf. Accessed February 12, 2018.

39. Caplan AL. Challenging teenagers' right to refuse treatment. Virtual Mentor 2007; 9(1):56–61.
40. Virginia Acts of Assembly 2007 Session. Chapter 597: an act to amend and reenact § 63.2–100 of the Code of Virginia, relating to abused or neglected children. 2007. Available at: http://leg1.state.va.us/cgi-bin/legp504.exe?071+ful+CHAP0597. Accessed February 27, 2018.
41. Ross LF. Against the tide: arguments against respecting a minor's refusal of efficacious life-saving treatment. Camb Q Healthc Ethics 2009;18(3):302–15 [discussion: 315–22].
42. Kopelman LM. The best-interests standard as threshold, ideal, and standard of reasonableness. J Med Philos 1997;22(3):271–89.
43. Diekema DS. Revisiting the best interest standard: uses and misuses. J Clin Ethics 2011;22(2):128–33.
44. Rhodes R, Holzman IR. Is the best interest standard good for pediatrics? Pediatrics 2014;134(Suppl 2):S121–9.
45. Online etymology dictionary: consent. 2001-2008. Available at: https://www.etymonline.com/word/consent. Accessed February 27, 2018.
46. Talati ED, Lang CW, Ross LF. Reactions of pediatricians to refusals of medical treatment for minors. J Adolesc Health 2010;47(2):126–32.
47. Doig C, Burgess E. Withholding life-sustaining treatment: are adolescents competent to make these decisions? Can Med Assoc J 2000;162(11):1585–8.
48. Khatibi M, Sheikholeslami R. Greenberger psychosocial maturity model: a brief review. J Educ Manage Stud 2016;6(2):57–61.
49. Feudtner C, Walter JK, Faerber JA, et al. Good-parent beliefs of parents of seriously ill children. JAMA Pediatr 2015;169(1):39–47.
50. Bluebond-Langner M. The private worlds of dying children. Princeton (NJ): Princeton University Press; 1978.

Children's Artwork
Its Value in Psychotherapy in Pediatric Palliative Care

Barbara M. Sourkes, PhD

KEYWORDS

- Pediatric palliative care • Life-threatening illness • Bereavement • Psychological
- Psychotherapy • Art techniques • Children • Adolescents

KEY POINTS

- Psychological care is a critical component of comprehensive pediatric palliative care, both during the illness and into bereavement.
- Children living with life-threatening illness and their siblings, as well as children of ill parents, face extraordinary psychological challenges.
- Psychotherapy affords a safe structure within which children can explore and contain the intensity of the overwhelming threat, and thus attain a measure of control.
- Structured art techniques can be powerful for children who are dealing with life-and-death realities, ineffable experiences for which words are often inadequate, even for adults.
- Rationale, instructions and examples of 3 structured art techniques are presented.

INTRODUCTION
Pediatric Palliative Care

Pediatric palliative care, still a new and emerging field, includes treatment for children and adolescents living with complex chronic and life-threatening conditions. It is an

Disclosure Statement: Nothing to declare.

Portions of this article are excerpted and adapted from The Deepening Shade: Psychological Aspects of Life-Threatening Illness, by Barbara M. Sourkes, © 1982, and from Armfuls of Time: The Psychological Experience of the Child with a Life-Threatening Illness, by Barbara M. Sourkes, © 1995, both by permission of the University of Pittsburgh Press.

In general, the term "children" is used to denote both children and adolescents unless a reference is specific to an adolescent.

The phrase "mental health professional" refers primarily to child/pediatric psychologists and psychiatrists, although other professions certainly may be included.

Stanford University School of Medicine, Division of Pediatric Critical Care Medicine, 770 Welch Road, Suite 435, Palo Alto, CA 94304-5876, USA

E-mail address: bsourkes@stanford.edu

Child Adolesc Psychiatric Clin N Am 27 (2018) 551–565
https://doi.org/10.1016/j.chc.2018.05.004
1056-4993/18/© 2018 Elsevier Inc. All rights reserved.

childpsych.theclinics.com

active and total approach (physical, psychological, social, and spiritual) that focuses on the following:

- Quality of life for the child and support for the family, with a particular focus on the healthy siblings
- Decision-making/establishment of goals of care for the child
- Management of symptoms
- Provision for respite

Importantly, the care extends from the time of diagnosis through the occurrence of the child's death and into bereavement. This arc may extend over many years.[1]

This definition provides the context for understanding the experience of children living with illness, both the patients and the healthy siblings. Children who have a parent who is ill typically fall into the world of adult palliative care; however, they are included in this discussion.

Psychotherapy

I felt much better because I knew that I had somebody to talk to all the time. Every boy needs a psychologist! To see his feelings!
(6-year-old-child, in isolation for stem cell transplantation)[2]

When we first went to the psychologist, my little brother thought she was a checkup doctor. But I explained to him: "You know how we lost our older sister? This doctor tries to get the sadness out of your heart." (7-year-old bereaved child)[3]

All these children, patients, siblings, children of ill parents, face inordinate psychic challenges that test their resilience to the utmost. Psychotherapy, the treatment modality unique to the mental health professional, reveals poignant and profound truths as children seek to integrate, or reintegrate, the shattered facets of their life. Through words, drawings, and play, children convey the experience of living with loss, either its lurking threat or the actuality, in an attempt to transform the essence of their reality into expression. Most children enter psychotherapy because of the stress engendered by the illness or the loss of a close loved one, rather than because of more general intrapsychic or interpersonal concerns.[4] The framework of psychotherapy affords a safe structure within which children can explore and contain the intensity of the overwhelming threat, and thus attain a measure of control.

Children's Artwork in Psychotherapy

Art techniques can be powerful in facilitating children's expression and their working through of complex emotions. This is especially true for children who are dealing with life-and-death realities, ineffable experiences for which words are often inadequate, even for adults. Structured art techniques allow the mental health professional to ask highly focused questions, rather than the broad queries more typical of psychotherapeutic interchange. Furthermore, by using drawings as an intermediary, these questions can often be posed earlier in the therapeutic process. Importantly, by asking children to draw in response to a specific question, the possibility that they will then provide a verbal explanation is enhanced. In this way, the interpretation of a given image is based within the child's psychic reality, and provides a foundation from which the psychotherapy can build. Of course, valuable disclosures also emerge from children's spontaneous artwork.

This article provides the rationale and instructions for several structured art techniques that the author has adapted for children facing illness and bereavement. The techniques include the following:

1. Mandala (color-feeling wheel)
2. Change-in-Family drawing
3. "Scariest" image

The children and adolescents whose images and explanations are shown include those living with life-threatening illness and their healthy siblings, children living with a parent who is ill, and bereaved children (who have lost either a sibling or a parent).

STRUCTURED ART TECHNIQUES
Mandala (Color-Feeling Wheel)

The mandala, a graphic symbolic pattern or design in the form of a circle, originated in Eastern religions. Jung believed that a mandala could mirror the state of the inner self.[5] The mandala is used in art therapy today, when a person is asked to fill in a blank circle to reflect "how you are feeling now." The author developed a more structured version of this projective technique, in the belief that a blank circle could be threatening to a child who is already overwhelmed by life-threatening illness or loss. The structured version gives them a scaffolding for their response. The steps in the structured version of mandala are described as follows.[4]

Definition of topic
The mental health professional defines a topic around which the mandala will be focused; for example, "How I felt when I heard my diagnosis" or "How I felt when my sibling/parent died."

Guided visualization (following is a general "script")
"Close your eyes and think about the day you were diagnosed/when your sibling or parent died... Remember where you were (hospital, doctor's office, clinic), who was with you, who told you and what words were used, what you saw... Remember how you felt... Open your eyes."

Some children find the visualization extremely anxiety-provoking. Clinical judgment is necessary as to whether to encourage the child to continue (perhaps with eyes open) or simply to omit this step. The visualization sets the stage for the concrete task that follows.

Array of feelings
"Now I am going to give you the names of feelings that other children have told me they felt when they heard the diagnosis/when their brother or sister or parent died. I want you to think about each feeling and see if it fits for you."

An array of feelings that are commonly attributed to the experience is presented. Each feeling should be written on a separate blank card and arranged randomly on the table to avoid the order bias of a vertical list. Some feelings for these topics might include, for example, shock, scared/terrified, sad, angry/mad, lonely, overwhelmed, guilty, ashamed, pain, confused, proud, hopeful. A category called "other feelings" also should be included. It is best to limit the number of feelings to approximately 8; by including "other feelings" children always have the option of adding more. The professional then gives the child a set of bright colored markers and a sheet of paper with a blank circle.

Color-feeling match and proportion
Now, choose a color to match each feeling. I want you to color in a part of the circle for each feeling. If the feeling was big, then make it a big part of the circle; if it was small, color in a small area (proportion). You may use the same color for more than one feeling as long as you label it clearly. If you had other feelings that I have not mentioned, put them in. When you are all finished, we can talk about the feelings and the colors you have chosen.

Title
Sometimes, before the discussion, I ask the child to give a title to their mandala. "This mandala/color-feeling circle is a story. If you had written your story as a book, it would have a title. Think of a title for your circle."

Because the mandala requires little time and minimal exertion or coordination, it can be used even with a child who is very ill. It also can be effective with very young children by reducing the number of feelings offered and reading them/discussing them aloud. Most children find the technique nonthreatening and enjoyable, and often express relief at having an array of feelings already articulated for them. Interpretation of the mandala is based on the child's choice of feelings, colors, proportions, order, overall design, and verbal associations. At its simplest, the mandala is a tool for facilitating expression; at its most complex, it is powerful in its symbolism and depth.

How I felt when I heard that I had leukemia "When I heard that I had leukemia, I turned pale with shock. That's why I chose yellow, it's a pale color. Scared is red, for blood. I was scared of needles, of seeing all the doctors, of what was going to happen to me. I was MAD [black] about a lot of things: staying in the hospital, taking medicines, bone marrows, spinal taps, IVs, being awakened in the middle of the night. I was sad [purple] that I didn't have my toys and that I was missing out on everything. I chose blue for lonely because I was crying about not being at home and not being able to go outside. Green is for hope: getting better, going home, eating food from home, and seeing my friends" (**Fig. 1**).

This description of a mandala by an 8-year-old boy captures the immediacy of the response to the diagnosis of a life-threatening illness. He articulates the shock; the fear of everything from the concrete medical procedures to the sudden possibility of

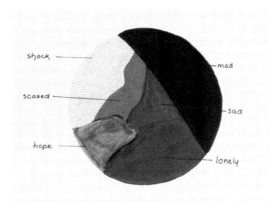

Fig. 1. How I felt when I heard that I had leukemia. (*Excerpted and adapted from* Armfuls of Time: The Psychological Experience of the Child with a Life-Threatening Illness, by Barbara M. Sourkes, © 1995, by permission of the University of Pittsburgh Press.)

an altered future ("what was going to happen to me"); the constellation of sadness, grief, and loneliness of separation; and the absence from his normal life. Accompanying all these feelings is a forthright statement of hope.[4]

The author had met with this child for 2 prior sessions without art materials, and he had been close to monosyllabic, answering every question with "it's okay I guess" or "not bad." He sat slumped, hiding most of his face under the visor of his baseball cap. Given the assigned mandala task, along with the offering of "other children's feelings," he communicated his experience thoughtfully and vividly.

Mixed messages A 10-year-old sibling spoke about her brother's diagnosis of a brain tumor: "*I feel scared (green), I feel as if I don't really know what is happening. Sad is blue, at first my parents just told me that my brother needed an operation. They didn't say it was cancer. Confused is yellow, just all mixed feelings, I don't know what to think. Hopeful is purple, bright, I don't really have a lot of hope, but maybe just a little. Angry is red because that is a mad color. Why him? What did it have to happen to him? My drawing is called 'Mixed Messages' because I have all of these different feelings and everyone is telling me different things. Like they say mostly that he is going to be okay, but they, and I, don't really believe it…*" (**Fig. 2**).[6]

My brother is really sick A 16-year-old adolescent included both depression and sadness in her mandala. This technique can be diagnostically useful in understanding adolescents' distinction between the virtually universal feelings of sadness/grief versus the symptom of depression (she decided to omit "shocked" because at the time of the drawing, she felt that the shock had worn off) (**Fig. 3**).

How I felt when I heard my brother had cancer: confused! "I was confused about everything. Not just the doctors' explanations, I GOT that information. I was confused about HOW this could have happened to my brother and to our family" (14-year-old girl). Of note is the fact that this adolescent had originally divided the circle into 3 segments, but "confused" took over everything. This mandala is instructive for the

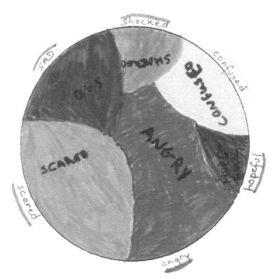

Fig. 2. Mixed messages. (*From* Pizzo PA, Poplack DG. Principles and Practice of Pediatric Oncology, 7th Edition. Philadelphia: Lippincott Williams and Wilkins; 2006; with permission.)

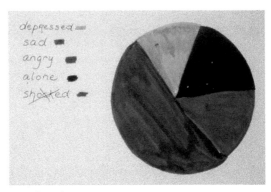

Fig. 3. My brother is really sick.

meaning of "confused": a word frequently used by children and family members. Medical teams often misinterpret the word as referring to cognitive confusion about "the facts" rather than a reaction of being completely overwhelmed and incredulous (**Fig. 4**).

My feelings about my dad's sickness A 12-year-old boy initially colored a wide, blue/black band in the circle and labeled it as "other feelings." He then added an extra blue/black "chunk" outside of the circle that he called "scared," a feeling he had not included in the original mandala. Once completed and on noting how these 2 areas comprised a large proportion of his feelings, he was able to articulate how truly terrified he felt (**Fig. 5**).

Mad (fâché) and furious (furieux) This 7-year-old child aggressively "attacked" the paper with his pens, using only brown and black, the 2 darkest colors, to depict his rage that overwhelmed any other feelings, and most certainly kept his profound sadness and anticipatory grief at bay. His only comment was: "That's all, I'm just mad (fâché) and furious (furieux) that my mom is sick" (**Fig. 6**).

It was like nothing, nothing... A 16-year-old girl reflected on the death of her younger brother: "The white space is for relief. My grandmother told me of his death. It was like nothing, nothing...He had been in a coma for months and getting bags of morphine 3 times a day... I used yellow and orange for shock because bright colors are like

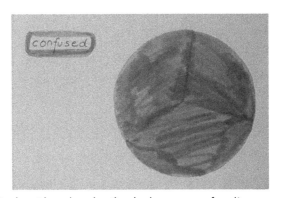

Fig. 4. How I felt when I heard my brother had cancer: confused!

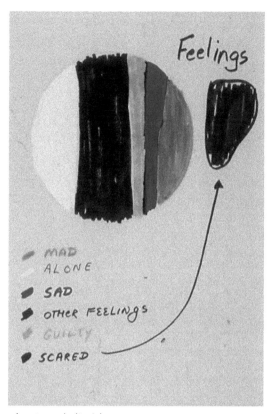

Fig. 5. My feelings about my dad's sickness.

shock." She also included sad and anger. The girl describes the paradox of death following the absence of a long coma: on the one hand, it is an empty "nothing"; on the other hand, its finality comes as a shock (**Fig. 7**).

The last 2 weeks were bad, really bad... A 12-year-old boy whose father had recently died said only: "The last 2 weeks were bad, really bad...." There is a lot of agitated

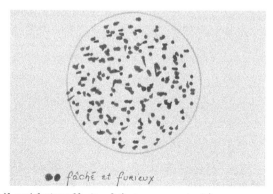

Fig. 6. Mad [fâché] and furious [furieux] that my mom is sick.

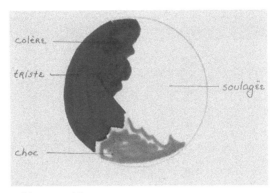

Fig. 7. It was like nothing...nothing.

movement and flow in his mandala. Shock (blue) and sad (purple) are somewhat similar colors; the blackness of relief stands out and is emphasized by his statement. The boy had witnessed and experienced inordinate suffering during those last 2 weeks, and through the mandala, he was able to admit to feeling relieved it was over (**Fig. 8**).

Change-In-Family Drawing

The Kinetic Family Drawing[7] has historically been a widely used art therapy technique. Children are asked to draw a picture of their entire family, and to show each member engaged in an activity. The drawing is then analyzed for factors including children's perceptions of their position within the family, the nature of the relationships, and the activities represented. The author has added another step to this technique. After the child has completed the basic family portrait, the child is asked: "What changed in your family after you got sick? Show the change in your drawing, either in picture or in words."[4] The responses to this simple question are often dramatic. This technique can be adapted for siblings, or for bereaved children. ("Draw your family the way it was before your __ died. Now show in your drawing what is different.") In fact, the technique can be used for any "before and after" situation. For all children, a "shortcut" can be simply to ask them to draw what has changed since, for example, their own diagnosis or the death of a family member. If children are hesitant to engage in this

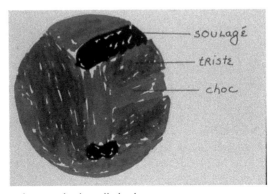

Fig. 8. The last 2 weeks were bad, really bad....

task, they can be encouraged simply to draw stick figures. Although the richness of individual representation is lost, the dynamics of the family system nonetheless emerge.

I didn't include myself

A 9-year-old boy (the patient) portrayed his older brother as a rock singer, his mother cooking, another brother, his father, and his pet hamster. When asked what had changed after his diagnosis, he added tears to each person. With regard to the omission of himself he explained: "I didn't include myself, because at the time I was in the hospital, and didn't think I'd be back in the picture." The little hamster imprisoned in the cage may well be his symbolic self-representation. The boy graphically conveyed his own anticipatory grief as well as that of his family (**Fig. 9**).[4]

My mother and I were the only girls...

A 13-year-old girl reflected after the death of her mother: "I'm worried about being alone. Even though I still have my father and brothers, my mother and I were the only girls, and now it's just me." For this child, being left as "the only girl" in the family felt equivalent to "being alone." She portrayed only herself, not including her brothers or father in the picture. Her copious blue tears and matching blue dress attest to her profound missing and loneliness (**Fig. 10**).

"Scariest" Image

"Think of the scariest experience, thought, feeling, or dream that you have had since you became ill/your sibling or parent became ill/your sibling or parent died ... Draw it."[4]

Through this technique, children are encouraged to bring out the extreme fear, often the very image that they are most afraid to express. The drawings represent a blend of actual and imagined experiences and focus on visible signs of illness, medical procedures, being alone, and death. The patient experiences the illness both physically and emotionally through symptoms, changes in appearance and body image, and the intrusion of technology. Images of these traumatic aspects reverberate for the siblings (or children of ill parents) who witness them and may become a source of great distress because their experience often goes unacknowledged.

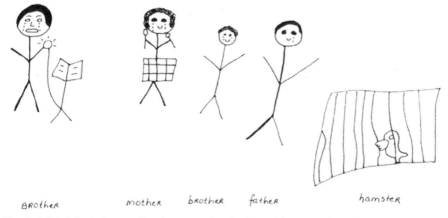

BROtheR   motheR   bRotheR   fatheR   hamsteR

Fig. 9. I didn't include myself.... (*Excerpted and adapted from* Armfuls of Time: The Psychological Experience of the Child with a Life-Threatening Illness, by Barbara M. Sourkes, Copyright 1995, by permission of the University of Pittsburgh Press.)

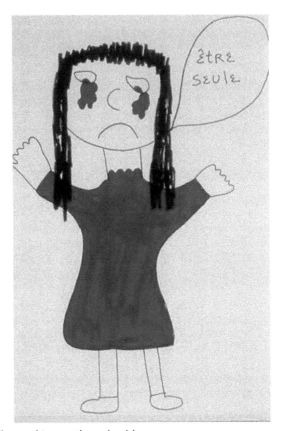

Fig. 10. My mother and I were the only girls.

I felt as if the IV was exploding in my arm
Psychologist: If you could choose 1 word to describe the scariest time since your diagnosis, what would it be?

Adolescent: PAIN: once I felt as if the IV was exploding in my arm! The boy went on to describe the excruciating pain he had felt amidst the chaos of his IV pole falling over and crashing to the floor. Note the horizontal arm at the bottom of drawing (**Fig. 11**).[6]

Dreaming of my sister in pain
In response to the question, "What is the scariest feeling, thought, or experience you have had since you sister became ill?" a child drew her response: "Dreaming of my sister in pain...." She depicted herself as a diminutive brown figure in a small bed, overwhelmed by the dream image of her sister in bright orange – screaming "OW" (**Fig. 12**).[6]

Scary cuts!
The 12-year-old boy who had described his feelings about "my dad's sickness" (see **Fig. 5**) did not hesitate when asked about his "scariest" image. His father's "scary cuts" were actually scars on his chest and abdomen from multiple surgeries, and the boy was traumatized whenever he saw them. It took many months of psychotherapy for him to realize that the transformation of "scary cuts" into scars represented healing and time passing from the acute illness (**Fig. 13**).

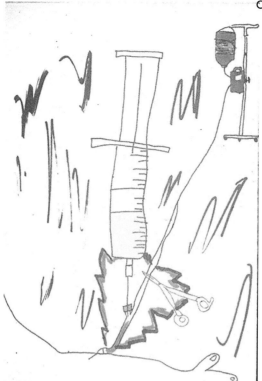

Fig. 11. I felt as if the IV was exploding in my arm. (*From* Sourkes B, Frankel L, Brown M, et al. Food, toys, and love: pediatric palliative care. Curr Probl Pediatr Adolesc Health Care 2005;35(9):365; with permission.)

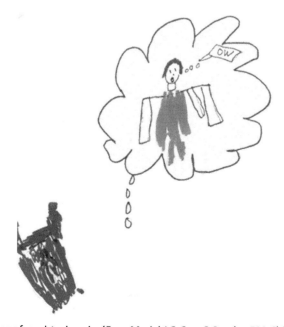

Fig. 12. Dreaming of my sister in pain. (*From* Muriel AC, Case C, Sourkes BM. Children's voices: the experience of patients and their siblings. In: Wolfe J, Hinds PS, Sourkes BM, editors. Textbook of interdisciplinary pediatric palliative care. Philadelphia: Saunders; 2011. p. 23; with permission.)

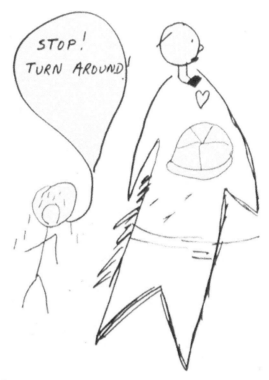

Fig. 13. Scary cuts!

Alone in the hospital

This 10-year-old child responded quickly to her "scariest" experience: being alone in the hospital. She lies in her bed in stark isolation, accompanied only by an ominous looking television.[4] The intensity of the aloneness is profound despite the almost constant presence of her parents (**Fig. 14**).

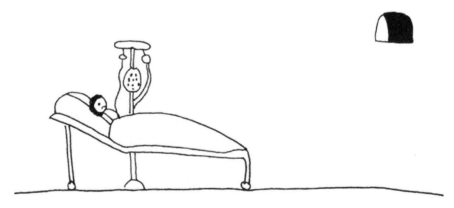

Fig. 14. Alone in the hospital. (*Excerpted and adapted from* Armfuls of Time: The Psychological Experience of the Child with a Life-Threatening Illness, by Barbara M. Sourkes, Copyright 1995, by permission of the University of Pittsburgh Press.)

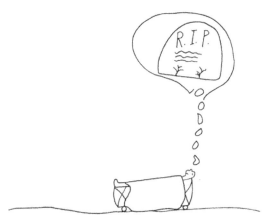

Fig. 15. "RIP": a patient's image. (*Excerpted and adapted from* Armfuls of Time: The Psychological Experience of the Child with a Life-Threatening Illness, by Barbara M. Sourkes, Copyright 1995, by permission of the University of Pittsburgh Press.)

"RIP" (rest in peace): patient and sibling

An 11-year-old boy portrayed himself lying in a hospital bed, the finality of death symbolized in his image of a tombstone with the initials "RIP."[4] In a "mirror-image," an 8-year-old sibling (not from the same family) drew his biggest fear: that his brother might die of his illness. Two faceless figures lower a coffin into the ground next to a tombstone inscribed "RIP" and a pile of dirt. Anxious scribbles filled part of the page (**Figs. 15** and **16**).[6]

I don't want to die (Je ne veux pas mourir)

An 8-year-old child who had recently lost her father said: "This is me telling my mother that I don't want to die. I am scared of death, especially in an airplane." Fears of harm and death in bereaved children may differ as to cause from their loved one's experience. In her picture, she has drawn her mouth in the shape of an airplane, thus fusing her words with the image of the fear (**Fig. 17**).

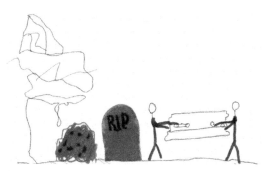

Fig. 16. "RIP": a sibling's image. (*From* Muriel AC, Case C, Sourkes BM. Children's voices: the experience of patients and their siblings. In: Wolfe J, Hinds PS, Sourkes BM, editors. Textbook of interdisciplinary pediatric palliative care. Philadelphia: Saunders; 2011. p. 25; with permission.)

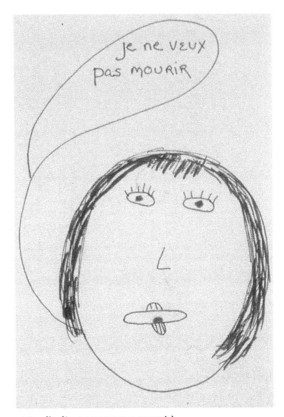

Fig. 17. I don't want to die (Je ne veux pas mourir).

SUMMARY

Although these structured art techniques are simple to administer, that "simplicity" is deceptive. As is evident in the clinical examples, they can evoke complex and powerful responses in children and adolescents. A cautionary note: as with any form of psychotherapy, there are risks when inexperienced or inadequately trained personnel undertake the work. They can unwittingly open up too much vulnerability too quickly without then knowing how to contain it. Within the world of pediatric palliative care and the exigencies of life-threatening illness and bereavement, this is an especially serious concern. Thus, these techniques are intended primarily for use within the context of psychotherapy, or with the consultation of mental health professionals when used in other settings.

REFERENCES

1. ACT (Association for Children with Life-threatening and Terminal Conditions and their families) and the RCOCH (Royal College of Paediatrics and Child Health). A Guide to the development of children's palliative care services. London (United Kingdom): 2003. p. 9.
2. Sourkes B. The deepening shade: psychological aspects of life-threatening illness. Pittsburgh (PA): University of Pittsburgh Press; 1982. p. 3.

3. Contro N, Kreicbergs U, Reichard W, et al. Anticipatory grief and bereavement. In: Wolfe J, Hinds P, Sourkes B, editors. Textbook of interdisciplinary pediatric palliative care. Philadelphia: Elsevier; 2011. p. 41–54.
4. Sourkes B. Armfuls of time: the psychological experience of the child with a life-threatening illness. Pittsburgh (PA): University of Pittsburgh Press; 1995. p. 3, 24, 31, 26, 35, 64, 114.
5. Fincher S. Creating mandalas. Boston (MA): Shambhala Press; 1991.
6. Muriel A, Case C, Sourkes B. Children's voices: the experience of patients and their siblings. In: Wolfe J, Hinds P, Sourkes B, editors. Textbook of interdisciplinary pediatric palliative care. Philadelphia: Elsevier; 2011. p. 18–29.
7. Burns R, Kaufman S. Kinetic family drawings. New York: Brunner-Mazel; 1970.

Parenting with a Life-Limiting Illness

Sarah E. Shea, PhD*, Cynthia W. Moore, PhD

KEYWORDS

- Parenting • Parental illness • Advanced cancer • Anticipated death • Bereavement
- Depression

KEY POINTS

- Parental illness confers risk for parental depression, impaired family functioning, and child adjustment difficulties.
- Parents often experience significant distress about the potential impact of their illness and anticipated death on children.
- When a parent's death is anticipated, clinicians have the opportunity to offer guidance that may mitigate risks to children, and reduce distress in parents.
- Clinical recommendations about communication about a parent's anticipated death, helping children spend meaningful time with an ill parent, and legacy leaving are provided.

INTRODUCTION

An estimated 10% of youth have a parent diagnosed with a serious medical illness, such as cancer, human immunodeficiency virus (HIV), hemophilia, multiple sclerosis (MS), Parkinson disease, or stroke,[1] and approximately 5% of children in Western countries experience parental loss before the end of their teenage years.[2] However, medical advances have helped many more patients manage life-threatening and life-limiting illnesses as chronic illnesses, affording parents more time with their young children. However, this also suggests that many dependent children witness a parent's medical treatment and advancing burdens of illness across longer portions of their childhoods. This article details some of the challenges of life-limiting parental illness, with a focus on advanced cancer, and offers clinically informed recommendations for supporting children's adjustment and emotional well-being as a parent nears end of life.

Disclosure: No disclosures.
Department of Psychiatry, Massachusetts General Hospital, Harvard Medical School, 55 Fruit Street, YAW 6900, Boston, MA 02114, USA
* Corresponding author.
E-mail address: Sshea6@mgh.harvard.edu

Child Adolesc Psychiatric Clin N Am 27 (2018) 567–578
https://doi.org/10.1016/j.chc.2018.05.002
childpsych.theclinics.com

WHEN PATIENTS ARE PARENTS, AND PARENTS ARE PATIENTS

Although difficult for anyone, patients facing a life-threatening illness who are also parenting dependent children contend with additional challenges. Parents with advanced cancer report struggling to balance the competing priorities of extending life and preserving functioning.[3] They are more likely to prioritize treatments that might extend lifespan over interventions designed to minimize pain and discomfort.[3,4] In addition, living with dependent children factors into patients' thinking about where to receive end-of-life care, given concerns about dying at home with children there.[3]

Just as being a parent creates unique challenges for patients, being a patient makes it harder to participate in usual social roles, including the role of parent. Parental role satisfaction and perceived parenting efficacy decrease after a cancer diagnosis in many ill parents as well as their partners,[5,6] with declines in parenting efficacy associated with reductions in the parent's availability and functioning, including more visits to a medical clinic, poorer health-related quality of life, and more depression and distress.[7]

However, individuals with chronic diseases are more likely to experience depression[8]; for example, HIV-positive mothers have been found to be at increased risk of depression relative to a comparison sample of uninfected mothers.[9] Among chronically ill patients, those with dependent children may be especially vulnerable to depression, because it has been reported that patients with advanced cancer with dependent children endorse higher levels of depression and anxiety than those without.[4] Increased depression among patients with dependent children may be related in part to increased parenting stress or the perception that the demands of child rearing are greater than the available resources with which to meet them.[10] Parents who rely on avoidance-based emotional regulation strategies to manage depression symptoms may be at increased risk for parenting stress.[11]

Specific awareness that an illness is life-limiting may further increase risk for depression. Among patients with newly diagnosed, incurable cancer, those who reported that they were terminally ill or who acknowledged that their oncologist's treatment goal was not to cure their cancer, had worse quality of life and more symptoms of depression and anxiety.[12] Awareness of having an incurable disease also heightens parenting concerns[13] and specifically raises the deeply painful worry about how children would cope should the parent die.

THE IMPACT OF PARENTAL ILLNESS ON CHILDREN

Between 15% and 30% of children coping with chronic parental illness experience internalizing symptoms such as depressed and anxious mood and intrusive thoughts and are also at risk for externalizing problems, irritability, somatic complaints, and academic and social difficulties.[1,14–19] Like their parents, children describe a range of concerns about the parent's illness. Latency-aged children report guilt, fears about the parent's symptoms, fear about the potential for the parent's death, and worry about the well parent. Adolescents also report guilt as well as empathy for the ill parent, concerns about household responsibilities, and problems with the relationship with parents.[20,21]

Increased recognition of the negative impacts of parental illness on children's adjustment has prompted investigation of potential mechanisms by which these effects are generated. It has been posited that serious chronic illness in parents negatively affects children's adjustment by disrupting family functioning, including role distribution, communication, family cohesion, and conflict.[22,23] Children's risk for poor adjustment outcomes may be further exacerbated when parental medical illness co-occurs with parental depression. In families in which a parent has cancer[24] or MS,[25] parental depression is associated with impaired family functioning and parenting behaviors, as well as child internalizing and externalizing problems. This finding is consistent with a broad body of literature linking depression and parenting stress to maladaptive parenting practices, characterized by lower levels of psychological availability, supervision, and consistent discipline and increased conflict and use of harsh and coercive parenting tactics, which in turn are associated with child adjustment problems.[11,26–28] More research is needed to better understand the links between child outcomes and parental depression and stress, family functioning, and parenting practices.

UNIQUE FACETS OF ANTICIPATED PARENTAL LOSS: CHALLENGES AND OPPORTUNITIES FOR INTERVENTION

The interplay of prognostic awareness, parental depression, parenting practices, and children's functioning described earlier suggests that children who recognize the parent's illness as terminal may be at particularly high risk for adjustment difficulties. Saldinger and colleagues[29] critiqued the existing literature on childhood bereavement for having largely overlooked the traumatic aspects of illness and dying in the service of promoting the maintenance of ties between the dying parent and child. Their qualitative study of 58 parentally bereaved children, aged 6 to 16 years, interviewed 8 to 36 months after a parent's death, suggested that many experienced a guilty tension between wanting and not wanting to see a dying parent. Parents did not always recognize children's distress, partly because children shielded them, and struggled to make decisions about how much children should be exposed to the dying parent.

Levels of psychiatric symptoms can also demonstrate the impact of anticipated deaths. A study comparing children aged 7 to 16 years with a terminally ill parent with a community control sample found that, before the death, children had more symptoms of depression and anxiety, whereas, by 7 to 12 months after the death, levels of symptoms were similar between groups. Thus the period of time during which a parent's illness is known to be terminal may be a time of high psychological vulnerability for children, even more than the period after the loss.[30]

There are mixed results regarding whether an anticipated death leads to worse postdeath outcomes than other losses. A study of 63 children, aged 3 to 13 years, who had lost a parent in the previous 6 months and their 38 surviving caregivers found that those whose loss followed a prolonged illness showed higher levels of maladaptive grief and posttraumatic stress symptoms, compared with children who experienced a sudden natural death (eg, heart attack).[31] Another study of 360 parent-bereaved children, aged 6 to 17 years, and their surviving parents, interviewed during the first 2 years following the death, found children's levels of depression were higher than nonbereaved community controls but lower than a clinically depressed group. Anticipation of death was not associated with worse outcomes but surviving parents' depression was.[32] Although there is still much to be learned about the unique effects of anticipated death, clinicians should be aware of the potential for heightened risk for symptoms of anxiety, maladaptive grief, and depression in children both before and after such a loss.

STRATEGIES TO SUPPORT COPING WITH ANTICIPATED PARENTAL LOSS

The gap between our evidence base and patients' questions and needs drives research but can also make it difficult for clinicians who value evidence-based practice to respond to these questions. That witnessing a parent's decline is intensely painful for all family members does not surprise patients in this situation, whose questions often focus on whether there are known ways to mitigate this risk. Both authors provide parent guidance consultations to adults through the Parenting At a Challenging Time (PACT) program at the Massachusetts General Hospital Cancer Center (**Box 1** provides program information) and thus regularly face the dilemma of responding as best we can to questions without easy answers. Three common challenges raised in consultations by parents with advanced cancer are described later, including relevant research findings, and ways that clinicians might navigate these challenges with the patients they serve are suggested. They are how to talk about anticipated death with children, how to help children spend meaningful time with the ill parent, and how to capitalize on the potential benefits of knowing death is imminent to promote positive grieving through legacy leaving.

TALKING ABOUT ANTICIPATED DEATH WITH CHILDREN

Parents with advanced cancer often find it challenging to respond to children's questions and concerns,[33] and some report that counselors are not adequately attuned to their specific needs and wish they could provide ideas about how other parents answered questions about parental death.[34] Many parents presenting for PACT consultations struggle to share with children news that active treatment is no longer possible or that a parent may die soon. At this point, parents often perceive that the primary challenge in talking to children is to describe next steps in a way that is realistic but leaves room for hope, even as they themselves grapple with what to hope for.

Are There Benefits to Open Communication?

Some children prefer that parents speak honestly about their health and treatment, and mention reluctance to upset parents by asking questions as an obstacle to talking openly.[33] Bereaved adolescents almost universally believe they should have been told that a parent was going to die within hours or days, but slightly less than 60% said that they themselves had been told this. Strikingly, 43% of them had not realized that the death was imminent, even just a few hours before it occurred.[35]

A small body of literature suggests potential benefits to open parent-child communication about a parent's cancer, including less anxiety, distress, intrusive thoughts,

---

Box 1
Parenting at a Challenging Time program

What: the Marjorie E. Korff PACT program provides support to adults served by our cancer center. Information about children's temperaments, developmental stages, and baseline functioning inform recommendations to parents. A variety of parent concerns are addressed, such as communicating with children about new diagnoses or advanced illness, and many end-of-life concerns.

Who: child-trained psychiatrists, psychologists, and social workers draw on their knowledge of normative child development, effective parenting practices, and child mental health.

Where: consultations occur in outpatient and inpatient areas of the hospital as well as by phone when face-to-face visits are not feasible.

When: patients are contacted within 24 hours of referral and many can be seen the same day. Depending on need, some meet once with a PACT clinician, and others meet multiple times.

How: referral sources include oncology and palliative care physicians, nurses, and social workers as well as patients themselves.

efforts to avoid thinking about the illness, and externalizing behaviors.[23,36–38] Children with only partial information about a parent's MS had more social problems and internalizing behaviors than children with either no information or full information (appropriate to developmental stage), hinting perhaps that children whose parents felt compelled to say something by virtue of observable symptoms, but were not really comfortable discussing the illness, had the hardest time.[39] The risks and benefits of open communication to children may vary depending on disease. For instance, the literature on parental HIV offers conflicting findings on the benefit of parental disclosure of serostatus. Children whose mothers disclosed their HIV status displayed lower levels of aggressiveness and negative self-esteem compared with children whose mothers had not disclosed in 1 study,[40] but higher levels of negative self-esteem, interpersonal problems, negative moods, and depression in 2 others.[9,41] However, none of these studies addressed explicit communication about the likelihood that a parent could die.

Finding a Way to Talk

Although much is still unclear about how sharing explicit information about a parent's impending death affects children, PACT consultations focus on open communication as a tool to help parents address children's specific worries, correct misconceptions, and model approach-based coping. In supporting parents to talk about the transition to end-of-life care with children, the authors start by assessing what parents think their children already understand, and then, based on the parents' values and willingness to be open, determining what needs to be shared. In some families, parents believe that children are unaware of the "big picture" and may strongly prefer that it stay that way. Children may, in fact, be as shielded as parents hope, but they may also be far more aware than parents realize and working hard to protect parents from their reactions.[29,33] In other families, parents assume that children recognize where the illness trajectory is leading ("She's smart, she gets it"), whereas in fact the children have not been able to extrapolate from the information they have to comprehension of this bigger picture. Children's understanding can be limited when parents have not shared enough information with them, when abstract thinking skills are limited by their developmental stage, and when the emotional content of the information makes processing its meaning difficult.

When the medical team has suggested that a patient's health status could decline soon but adults are reluctant to talk with their children about this, clinicians may be faced with a complicated mix of multiple family members' needs and preferences. For example, a coparent may struggle with wanting to respect the patient's more gradual acceptance of prognosis but feel concerned about children's adjustment to difficult changes for which they may be unprepared. In contrast, an ill parent may be dissuaded from talking more openly by family members providing more of children's day-to-day care who worry that children would "fall apart" if they learned about the severity of the illness. Sometimes the adults are united in their belief that the best way to protect children is to avoid talking about the illness, and the medical team is left holding the anxiety that children are unprepared.

In these cases, naming the different points of view, exploring and testing the beliefs that inform them, and helping parents recognize new aspects of their children's experience can be helpful. Clinicians may, for example, share the perspective that shielding children too much can have unintended consequences, such as the child's being unprepared for and shocked by a loss, feeling lied to, or missing an opportunity to say goodbye to the parent that the child might have wanted. Sometimes simply raising the question of whether children might be already wondering about whether the parent will survive leads to a parent's recognizing (or acknowledging) that the child has signaled concern. Then, parents can be encouraged to imagine how it might feel to the child to have that worry but not feel able to talk about it. Sometimes a description of worries expressed by other same-age children sparks a moment of recognition in a patient that their child, too, might have concerns. For instance, sharing that some adolescents imagine that, if a parent were to die, there would be severe financial impacts; whether this is true or not, reducing uncertainty by talking about it may allow teens to use more problem-focused coping strategies and to feel more confident that they and other family members could cope.

For parents who are willing to talk directly with children about the likelihood of death but feel stuck on the mechanics of the conversation, conversational guidelines can be helpful (**Table 1**). It is important to help parents find ways to check in with children throughout the process of sharing new information to ensure that they have accurately gauged children's understanding. In addition, although parents recognize that choosing what words to use is important, they may be less aware of other elements

Table 1 Communication guide for sharing bad news with children	
Talking Points	**Words to Try**
Invite children to share what they have noticed	• What have you been noticing about Mom's health since the last time we talked?
Connect observations to new information	• You've seen that I've been in bed a lot lately, even in the daytime. That's because I have felt so, so tired • You know that Mom has been in the hospital for the last 5 nights
Review treatment course, linking observable aspects of parent's condition to information about the illness/progression as distinct from treatment side effects	• You might remember I've had a lot of visits to the doctor, to try to get better from cancer. Even though my doctors and I have tried hard, the cancer keeps getting worse. That's partly why I've been so tired • You know that I have tried a lot of different cancer treatments: chemotherapy, surgery, radiation. It's been hard, but I wanted to do everything I could to get better. I talked to my doctor yesterday and learned that the cancer has again gotten worse. That helps explain why I've been so tired lately: it's not just side effects from the medicine like before, it's that the cancer has spread
Describe what is next: prognosis, short-term changes	• My doctors told me that there aren't any other treatments they think will slow down the cancer/make me any better/help me live longer • At this point, Dad may not be able to live much longer. His doctors told us he could die in as little as a few days. If you want to spend time with him, let's find a way for you to do it soon
Describe current hopes	• Now I will take medicine just to make sure I am not in pain. I'll be [where?] and have [who?] helping take care of me. I will focus on enjoying each day as much as I can

of their communication style that influence children's reactions. For example, parents' reactions to children's negative emotions, and ability to communicate about these emotions, relates to children's use of constructive coping strategies.[42] Helping parents realistically consider the impact of their own emotions on children and children's likely emotional reactions to information, and being gently curious about how they usually comfort children and how children respond to that, are additional elements of our parent guidance consultations.

SPENDING TIME TOGETHER NEAR END OF LIFE/SAYING GOODBYE

Many families intuitively find meaningful ways to be together during the end stages of an illness: sharing stories, looking at pictures, talking about everyday life, expressing love in familiar ways. Some families have a harder time managing this and may be ambivalent about how much to encourage children to spend time with a dying parent versus maintaining the routine. Some parents hold clear opinions about whether time with the dying parent is beneficial or not, whereas others attempt to follow the child's lead by giving the child control through choices. Although helpful to an extent, children who feel unsupported in choosing their preferred level of contact with an ill parent may feel burdened by this responsibility, or torn between guilt at not spending time with the ill parent or saying goodbye and fear or sadness around being exposed to a parent's physical and/or emotional suffering.

Rather than prescribing anything, it may help to guide parents to consider what their family style has always been, what is gained and lost by each family member by spending more time with the dying parent, and whether there are creative ways of meeting individual needs (**Box 2**). For example, for more sensitive or emotionally reactive children, or children who express reluctance to witness parental decline, plans can be made for the child to connect to the dying parent through phone calls, texts

---

Box 2
Supporting children's time with a parent near end of life

- Do not assume that no overt reaction equals no reaction to parent's decline
  - Suggest to child that changes may be distressing
  - Normalize a range of reactions to impending death, including wishes to avoid witnessing suffering and physical changes

- When making decisions about visits, consider each child's temperament, especially emotional intensity and sensitivity to stimuli (visual, olfactory, auditory) and others' emotions
  - Offer choices, with guidance
  - Normalize child's wish not to miss out on usual activities that help the child feel capable, confident, connected to peers
  - Continue to renegotiate comfortable balance of time with family, peers, and passions

- Consider relative benefits of physical distance versus closeness between the child and the dying parent and explore ways to protect the child from distress
  - Closeness to parent may bring: reassurance of mutual love; comfort from a parent (particularly one who is able to talk about the grief process); connection to extended family; child's pleasure or pride in bringing a parent happiness by visiting but also increased chance of witnessing graphic stimuli that put child at risk for posttraumatic stress symptoms
  - Distance from the parent may bring: the comfort and predictability of everyday routines; the sense of mastery that comes from regular engagement in school and activities; easier access to social support from peers; more opportunities for distraction to help with emotion regulation but also potential for guilt, especially if siblings made a different choice; worry the parent will not appreciate the child's love

to be read by other family members, or sending artwork or other tokens of love. Children who will be spending time with a parent nearing end of life can be prepared somewhat with a description of what they are likely to see and hear. It is helpful as well for a trusted adult to check in with the child after a visit about what the child noticed and whether anything was surprising or particularly upsetting.

Sometimes children are reluctant to visit for reasons other than worry about seeing the parent's decline. Rather than assuming the child feels frightened, if parents can uncover these concerns, sometimes they can be addressed. Common concerns include feeling that other people will intrude on the child's wished-for time alone with the parent, embarrassment about crying in front of other family or staff, feeling like they do not know what to say or do in the room, and feeling physically confined by a small space.

LEGACY LEAVING

When a parent's death is anticipated, families can take steps to bolster bonds between ill parents and their children, and cultivate a lasting connection that will remain after the parent dies. One primary channel through which this is achieved is legacy leaving. Legacy has been defined as a "process of passing one's self through generations, creating continuity from the past through the present to the future."[43] In our clinical work, the authors encourage families to conceive of legacy leaving as an intergenerational gift. For ill parents, legacy leaving offers a chance to make meaning of their own lives. For instance, a qualitative study of adult women found that participants of varying ages emphasized legacy leaving as a means to pass on elements of themselves, such as identity, values, beliefs, and family and cultural history, and that this issue was especially salient among those with life-threatening illnesses.[44] Legacy leaving may also be particularly affirming for ill parents by allowing them to contribute to their children's adjustment to bereavement.

However, preparing legacy gifts is inherently difficult work, often fraught with mixed feelings for parents. It requires contact with and acceptance of painful internal experiences, including thoughts and emotions elicited by the reality of impending death, lost time spent parenting, and the permanent separation from children. Not surprisingly, the prospect of preparing legacy gifts can feel overwhelming for parents and their partners, and, in the context of so many other illness-related and parenting-related challenges, it is understandable that some may shy away from, or struggle to initiate, the process. Clinical experience suggests that ill parents benefit from support with legacy leaving, both from family members and professionals. This work can be completed incrementally over time, affording the ill parent an opportunity for emotional pacing during the process.

Parents can benefit from specific, concrete suggestions about the varied forms that legacy leaving can take; this context helps parents imagine how they might authentically tailor their legacy gifts. Some parents choose to set aside, or allow a child to select, a material item as part of their legacy. In a qualitative, community sample of parentally bereaved children, two-thirds of the participants reported using objects they associated with their deceased parents as a strategy to maintain shared memories and connections.[45] Select items sometimes include a favorite or frequently used belonging, such as a signature head scarf, cozy sweater, or blanket. Other belongings, such as a piece of jewelry, furniture, or family heirloom, can be meaningful as well. This process can be done either as the parents approach end of life or shortly after their deaths, and can serve as a comforting link to a parent in the wake of the parent's death and beyond.

Legacy leaving also affords an opportunity to preserve memories for children, providing a tool through which children can rehearse memories in the future. For instance, annotated scrapbooks or photograph albums can archive family stories. Some relics can serve the dual purpose of capturing an existing family tradition as well as conveying valuable stories from generations past. For instance, in passing on her grandmother's candlesticks, a mother could share fond memories of holidays spent with her children along with memories of childhood holidays spent with her grandparents. Gifts can also maintain religious or cultural traditions, such as a religious text or recipe book.

Legacy gifts offer a powerful and lasting reminder for children that they were deeply known and loved by their deceased parent. Through letter writing, for example, parents can encapsulate some of their favorite memories of each child, and highlight for their child the distinguishing qualities that make them unique. Some parents choose to leave letters, cards, or other items to correspond with future developmental milestones, such as birthdays, graduations, or marriages. Broad messages that emphasize overarching values (eg, curiosity of learning) rather than specific goals (eg, graduation from medical school) may be most helpful. Parents should ensure that legacy gifts are roughly equal for all children in a family.

Children who have lost a parent, particularly when they are very young, may also appreciate strategies through which they can continue to get to know the deceased parent. Ill parents can prepare a library of their favorite books, movies, or songs, which can be very meaningful to bereaved children as they mature. Parents can also impart a "living legacy" to their children by recruiting a cohort of close family and friends who are eager to meet with children in an ongoing way as they grow up, and who can supply children with new memories through which they can come to know their parent more deeply. After a parent dies, surviving coparents can play a central role in upholding legacy and fostering connection to the deceased parent; for instance, by developing memorializing rituals and facilitating contact with the family of the deceased.[45]

SUMMARY

Parents with life-threatening illness face unique challenges in their dual roles as patients and parents. They are at risk for depression, parenting stress, and impaired family functioning, and their children are also at risk for adjustment difficulties. In addition to treatment of depression and other mental health issues, patients may also benefit from evidence-informed guidance addressing the challenges of parenting while ill. Consultations should be tailored to each family, with consideration of the developmental stage and temperament of children. Attention to communication about anticipated death, helping children spend meaningful time with an ill parent, and legacy leaving are recommended.

REFERENCES

1. Sieh DS, Visser-Meily JM, Meijer AM. Differential outcomes of adolescents with chronically ill and healthy parents. J Child Fam Stud 2013;22(2):209–18.

2. Høeg BL, Johansen C, Christensen J, et al. Early parental loss and intimate relationships in adulthood: a nationwide study. Dev Psychol 2018;54(5):963–74.

3. Check DK, Park EM, Reeder-Hayes KE, et al. Concerns underlying treatment preferences of advanced cancer patients with children. Psychooncology 2016; 26(10):1491–7.

4. Nilsson ME, Maciejewski PK, Zhang B, et al. Mental health, treatment preferences, advance care planning, location, and quality of death in advanced cancer patients with dependent children. Cancer 2009;115(2):399–409.

5. Siegel K, Raveis VH, Bettes B, et al. Perceptions of parental competence while facing the death of a spouse. Am J Orthopsychiatry 1990;60(4):567–76.

6. Cho OH, Yoo YS, Hwang KH. Comparison of parent-child communication patterns and parental role satisfaction among mothers with and without breast cancer. Appl Nurs Res 2015;28(2):163–6.

7. Moore CW, Rauch PK, Baer L, et al. Parenting changes in adults with cancer. Cancer 2015;121(19):3551–7.

8. Chapman DP, Perry GS, Strine TW. The vital link between chronic disease and depressive disorders. Prev Chronic Dis 2005;2(1):A14.

9. Brackis-Cott E, Mellins CA, Dolezal C, et al. The mental health risk of mothers and children: the role of maternal HIV infection. J Early Adolesc 2007;27(1): 67–89.

10. Abidin RR. Manual for the parenting stress index. Odessa (FL): Psychological Assessment Resources; 1995.

11. Shea SE, Coyne LW. Maternal dysphoric mood, stress, and parenting practices in mothers of head start preschoolers: the role of experiential avoidance. Child Fam Behav Ther 2011;33(3):231–47.

12. Nipp RD, Greer JA, El-Jawahri A, et al. Coping and prognostic awareness in patients with advanced cancer. J Clin Oncol 2017;35(22):2551–7.

13. Muriel AC, Moore CW, Baer L, et al. Measuring psychosocial distress and parenting concerns among adults with cancer: the parenting concerns questionnaire. Cancer 2012;118(22):5671–8.

14. Grabiak BR, Bender CM, Puskar KR. The impact of parental cancer on the adolescent: an analysis of the literature. Psychooncology 2007;16(2):127–37.

15. Phillips F. Adolescents living with a parent with advanced cancer: a review of the literature: adolescents advanced parental cancer: review. Psychooncology 2014; 23(12):1323–39.

16. Visser A, Huizinga GA, Hoekstra HJ, et al. Emotional and behavioral functioning of children of a parent diagnosed with cancer: a cross-informant perspective. Psychooncology 2005;14(9):746–58.

17. Rainville F, Dumont S, Simard S, et al. Psychological distress among adolescents living with a parent with advanced cancer. J Psychosoc Oncol 2012;30(5): 519–34.

18. Krattenmacher T, Kuhne F, Fuhrer D, et al. Coping skills and mental health status in adolescents when a parent has cancer: a multicenter and multi-perspective study. J Psychosom Res 2013;74(3):252–9.

19. Siegel K, Mesagno FP, Karus D, et al. Psychosocial adjustment of children with a terminally ill parent. J Am Acad Child Adolesc Psychiatry 1992;31(2):327–33.

20. Christ GH, Siegel K, Freund B, et al. Impact of parental terminal cancer on latency-age children. Am J Orthopsychiatry 1993;63(3):417–25.

21. Christ GH, Siegel K, Sperber D. Impact of parental terminal cancer on adolescents. Am J Orthopsychiatry 1994;64(4):604–13.

22. Armistead L, Klein K, Forehand R. Parental physical illness and child functioning. Clin Psychol Rev 1995;15(5):409–22.

23. Watson M, St James-Roberts I, Ashley S, et al. Factors associated with emotional and behavioural problems among school age children of breast cancer patients. Br J Cancer 2006;94(1):43–50.

24. Schmitt F, Piha J, Helenius H, et al. Multinational study of cancer patients and their children: factors associated with family functioning. J Clin Oncol 2008;26: 5877–83.
25. Diareme S, Tsiantis J, Kolaitis G, et al. Emotional and behavioural difficulties in children of parents with multiple sclerosis: a controlled study in Greece. Eur Child Adolesc Psychiatry 2006;15(6):309–18.
26. Faulkner RA, Davey M. Children and adolescents of cancer patients: the impact of cancer on the family. Am J Fam Ther 2002;30(1):63–72.
27. Lorber MF, O'Leary SG, Kendziora KT. Mothers' overreactive discipline and their encoding and appraisals of toddler behavior. J Abnorm Child Psychol 2003; 31(5):485–94.
28. Krattenmacher T, Kühne F, Ernst J, et al. Parental cancer: factors associated with children's psychosocial adjustment–a systematic review. J Psychosom Res 2012; 72(5):344–56.
29. Saldinger A, Cain A, Porterfield K. Managing traumatic stress in children antici-pating parental death. Psychiatry 2003;66(2):168–81.
30. Siegel K, Karus D, Raveis VH. Adjustment of children facing the death of a parent due to cancer. J Am Acad Child Adolesc Psychiatry 1996;35(4):442–50.
31. Kaplow JB, Howell KH, Layne CM. Do circumstances of the death matter? Iden-tifying socioenvironmental risks for grief-related psychopathology in bereaved youth. J Trauma Stress 2014;27(1):42–9.
32. Cerel J, Fristad MA, Verducci J, et al. Childhood bereavement: psychopathology in the 2 years postparental death. J Am Acad Child Adolesc Psychiatry 2006; 45(6):681–90.
33. Kennedy VL, Lloyd-Williams M. Information and communication when a parent has advanced cancer. J Affect Disord 2009;114(1):149–55.
34. Turner J, Clavarino A, Yates P, et al. Development of a resource for parents with advanced cancer: what do parents want. Palliat Support Care 2007;5(2): 135–45.
35. Bylund-Grenklo T, Kreicbergs U, Uggla C, et al. Teenagers want to be told when a parent's death is near: a nationwide study of cancer-bereaved youths' opinions and experiences. Acta Oncol 2015;54(6):944–50.
36. Rosenheim E, Reicher R. Informing children about a parent's terminal illness. J Child Psychol Psychiatry 1985;26(6):995–8.
37. Lindqvist B, Schmitt F, Santalahti P, et al. Factors associated with the mental health of adolescents when a parent has cancer. Scand J Psychol 2007;48(4): 345–51.
38. Huizinga GA, Visser A, Van Der Graaf WT, et al. The quality of communication be-tween parents and adolescent children in the case of parental cancer. Ann Oncol 2005;16:1956–61.
39. Paliokosta E, Diareme S, Kolaitis G, et al. Breaking bad news: communication around parental multiple sclerosis with children. Fam Syst Health 2009;27(1): 64–76.
40. Murphy DA, Steers WN, Dello Stritto ME. Maternal disclosure of mothers' HIV se-rostatus to their young children. J Fam Psychol 2001;15(3):441–50.
41. Murphy DA, Marelich WD, Hoffman D. A longitudinal study of the impact on young children of maternal HIV serostatus disclosure. Clin Child Psychol Psychiatry 2002; 7(1):55–70.
42. Gentzler AL, Contreras-Grau JM, Kerns KA, et al. Parent–child emotional communication and children's coping in middle childhood. Soc Dev 2005; 14(4):591–612.

43. Hunter EG, Rowles GD. Leaving a legacy: toward a typology. J Aging Stud 2005; 19(3):327–47.
44. Hunter EG. Beyond death: inheriting the past and giving to the future, transmitting the legacy of one's self. Omega 2007;56(4):313–29.
45. Saldinger A, Cain AC, Porterfield K, et al. Facilitating attachment between school-aged children and a dying parent. Death Stud 2004;28(10):915–40.

Bereavement After a Child's Death

Danielle Jonas, MSW, LCSW[a],*, Caitlin Scanlon, MSW[b], Rachel Rusch, MSW, MA[a],
Janie Ito, M.Div, BCC[c], Marsha Joselow, MA, MSW, LICSW[d]

KEYWORDS

- Parent bereavement • Sibling bereavement • Palliative care • Pediatrics • Grief
- Pediatric death • Provider grief • Memory making

KEY POINTS

- The death of a child can have an impact on various members of a child's family and community. Often this loss has the most direct impact on the child's primary caregivers, immediate family members, siblings, and peers. It may also have an impact on health care providers as well as additional members of the child's community, such as those within their school, church congregation, and peers.
- Grief after the death of a child can have an impact on bereavement in a multitude of ways, including spiritually, emotionally, developmentally, and functionally.
- Those who are experiencing grief after a pediatric death can receive support in their coping through a multitude of resources, such as individual/group counseling, online support groups, family/sibling camps, and bereavement follow-up provided by hospitals and/or hospices.
- Pediatric loss can also have an impact on providers, who and can benefit from supportive resources and opportunity for processing. It can be beneficial for hospitals and other institutions to offer standardized and individual support for providers. Palliative care teams, social workers, and chaplains can be helpful in offering resources and best practices in this regard.

The death of a child is often a heart-wrenching experience that can have a significant impact on parents, siblings, and families while also often having ripple effects throughout the child's community. Pediatric loss has an impact on family structure and dynamics, individual identity formation, and conceptualization as well as professional practice. This article explores bereavement after a child's death through the lens of the family, the parent, the sibling, the forgotten grievers, and the provider.

[a] Division of Comfort and Palliative Care, Children's Hospital Los Angeles, Los Angeles, CA, USA; [b] Integrated Care Management, Palliative Care Team, Riley Hospital for Children, Indiana University Health, Indianapolis, IN, USA; [c] Spiritual Care and Clinical Pastoral Education, Children's Hospital Los Angeles, Los Angeles, CA, USA; [d] Pediatric Advance Care Team, Boston Children's Hospital, Dana Farber Cancer Institute, Boston, MA, USA
* Corresponding author. 4650 Sunset Boulevard, #170, Los Angeles, CA 90027.
E-mail address: Daniellefayejonas@gmail.com

Child Adolesc Psychiatric Clin N Am 27 (2018) 579–590
https://doi.org/10.1016/j.chc.2018.05.010
1056-4993/18/© 2018 Elsevier Inc. All rights reserved.

FAMILY EXPERIENCE
Family Modeling of Emotional Processing

Children of any developmental stage may be acutely aware of the expression and processing of grief that surrounds them after their sibling has died. This is not to say that such emotions must be hidden or veiled; in fact, the allowance for parental experience of bereavement to be shared and reflected on openly can create a feeling of safety within a bereaved child who is learning how to navigate such an experience.[1] Just as grief, mourning, and bereavement take of many forms for parents throughout a lifetime, so do such navigations for bereaved siblings. Creating the space for honest and loving language, even when the words are imperfect and difficult to find, can at times be the most helpful intervention for a child whose sibling has died. Overall, the sense of connection that one is not alone in such an experience can be one of the most beneficial therapeutic supports.

Holidays/Anniversaries

Holidays and anniversaries can be especially challenging for bereaved families because they are so acutely reminded of the loved one who has died and the impact their absence has had on the family. Feelings of dread, worry, guilt, sadness, and avoidance may arise. Although it may be an emotional experience, it is imperative that children and families have the opportunity to remember and honor their loved one, not only at their death but also for years to come. Creating new family traditions on holidays, birthdays, and anniversaries can become special moments in which a family can continue on their bereavement journey. As a family reconstructs the meaning of their child's life and death, they can create lasting legacy through the addition of new ways to honor their child in the hopes of off-setting the potential of complicated grief.[2]

Although these special days can be a reminder of the pain and loss, ignoring them or pretending that they do not exist may be more detrimental to the family. The absence of acknowledgment can lead to feelings of isolation for individual family members. The emotions do not simply disappear but rather simmer until they are too much to bear. Although families may feel particularly vulnerable, they are honest expressions of the grief journey. If a family can work together to discuss how they will honor their loved ones or create new traditions, this can alleviate some of the stress that will be presented on the actual day.[3]

Amongst the tears and challenges, sharing memories and legacy can be comforting and cathartic for each family member. Still, parents/guardians should remain cognizant of the varying cognitive ages of surviving siblings. What causes emotional pain for one family member may bring pleasure to another. When family traditions arise, younger children are more apt to desire continuing previous traditions that involved the deceased, whereas older children and adolescents may feel it is too painful to continue the traditions while experiencing the memories of partaking in them with the deceased. Therefore, it may be especially helpful to offer choices for level of involvement of activities for each family member. Keeping open patterns of communication will assist in assessing and addressing each individual family member's needs.[3,4]

Above all, families should be reminded that it is okay to still experience joy around the holidays, despite the absence of their loved one. Over time, each family can work to develop their own traditions honoring their loved ones. As providers, it can be of service to the family to acknowledge these difficult days and develop plans to maximize support and anticipate disabling grief and anxiety.

PARENT EXPERIENCE
Spiritual Impact

Each person has a unique perspective on death, informed by their own religious/spiritual beliefs. A child coming to a hospital often causes emotional stress for the child and the family unit. If the patient/family identify as spiritual or religious, spiritual stressors can be exacerbated and can result in spiritual distress. The chaplaincy field recognizes that people who identify as religious or spiritual are interested in having spiritual needs addressed when hospitalized. For example, in recent studies, patients suffering from serious illness say that spirituality is important and would like a chaplain visit.[5,6] Additionally, when there are spiritual care visits to these patients and families, there is a direct correlation to improved patient/family satisfaction.[7] Nash and colleagues[8] define religious care versus spiritual care, as follows: "*Religious care* relates specifically to the tenets, practices, rituals and conventions of a particular religious faith...*Spiritual care* involves facilitating an individual's engagement with the existential questions of life, which involve identity, purpose and the potentiality of a relationship with or connectedness to a transcendent dimension or a sense of the sacred."[8]

In the United States, the experience of religion and spirituality is diverse and individualized. According to the Pew Research Center in a survey from November 2015, although Americans are becoming less religious, with 23% identifying as "religiously unaffiliated," in the same survey, 89% of Americans said they believed in God, and 77% identified with a religious faith. The study also cites an increase in spirituality in Americans.[9]

To optimize the spiritual and religious needs of patients/families at end of life and in bereavement, a thorough assessment of spiritual needs and coping strategies is imperative. Professional chaplains are trained to conduct an assessment that aims to delineate the needs of each individual family member. This experience is unique and often influenced by cultural and familial traditions. Particular rituals and practices, prayers, and final blessings are often a crucial part of end of life and bereavement and, therefore, it is incumbent on chaplains to assure that individual needs are assessed effectively.

Both helpful and unhelpful spiritual/religious beliefs, helpful beliefs deemed positive and unhelpful beliefs deemed negative by the effect that they have on the coping of the family.

Helpful beliefs are deemed positive by a family if they aide in coping. Negative beliefs are deemed negative by a family if they have a negative impact on coping. Examples are as follows:

- Buddhism: suffering is considered part of life that cannot be avoided.
- Hinduism: there is reincarnation.
- Christianity: there is hope of life after death; in many traditions, there is belief in continued life after death.

Religion/spirituality exists to help finding meaning in suffering and in finitude. Although traditions can be diverse, religion and spirituality are the human motivators in making meaning for existential questions of suffering and death. Those who are not particularly religious are still able to create a legacy for their child, through the use of meaning making as a positive coping tool in bereavement.

Unhelpful Spiritual Responses

Unhelpful spiritual beliefs are ones that cause spiritual suffering or spiritual distress. Parents who demonstrate spiritual struggle seem more isolated when/after the death occurs. Feelings of anger, abandonment by God, and guilt are often part of the spiritual process of bereavement and are normal. These become unhelpful when a bereaved individual is unable to process this experience. Often deeply religious friends or family members encourage parents to pray constantly and not give up, making promises that if they are faithful enough, God will heal their child. This unhelpful spiritual belief/support often causes major spiritual distress if a child dies and often negatively affects spiritual coping in bereavement.

Making meaning of a child's death is important to positive spiritual coping. Faith communities are often a strong source of support to patients and families as they move through their disease experience, end of life, and bereavement process. Often chaplains connect families with local faith communities at end of life and during the bereavement. Especially for family members who find religion an important aspect of their life, chaplains and clergy members can play a crucial role in providing support in bereavement.

Emotional Responses

Guilt

Guilt can most simply be defined as the emotional component of grief. It is most commonly manifested as regrets and self-blame and is often experienced by parents as they navigate their grief journey.[10] Families' minds frequently wander to the "what ifs" and "if onlys" as they grapple with the painful loss of their beloved child. It is natural and expected for families to experience these feelings and be riddled with questions.[4] Although is it natural to wonder about how a child's death could have been avoided, prevented, or prolonged, it is imperative to remind families that they are not to blame. At the same time, these feelings of guilt should be acknowledged as a real experience and it may be best for the family to speak with a psychosocial professional to assist in mitigating these emotions.

Self-blame

Self-blame is 1 of the 2 main components of parental guilt.[11] It is typically experienced as a result of a family member feeling that he or she has failed at the primary job of protecting a child due to a profound sense of accountability for the child's welfare.[12,13] Family members perceive that they were unable to keep the child safe and because of their actions, the child has died. This may reveal itself through questions such as, "What if I had found another doctor?" or "What if I had taken him to the doctor sooner?"[4]

Regret

Regret is the second of the 2 main components of parental guilt in bereavement.[11] When a family experiences regrets, they are often leading themselves to a belief that they could have done something differently in an effort to produce a better outcome. Additionally, it is a sense of unfinished business and the loss of future experiences with the deceased. Unlike self-blame, regret does not impair a sense of self.[11] A sense of regret may lead to questions, such as, "If only I had allowed him to be a part of the treatment conversations?" or "I wish I had thought about that being the last time I ever heard her voice."

In an effort to best assist in aiding families as they experience distressing guilt, providers can allow space for compassionate processing of the emotions. Providers should remain aware that although the experience of guilt in the short term is natural and normal, in the long term, it can be more concerning and has been shown a precursor for depression.[10,11]

Evolving perspectives/relationships
Parents' relationships with their children who have died continue to evolve for the rest of their lives, despite their physical absence. Depending on religious and cultural beliefs, families are likely to relate to their child in a variety of ways. Some parents report having spiritual or emotional experiences with their children, whereas others find peace in having their child's cremated remains in their home. Families may share narratives about their child's spirit being present for certain events or at specific times throughout the day.[4]

Parenting additional children
A significant challenge that is often reflected in the parental grief experience is the difficulty of navigating a parent's grief while also continuing to parent living children. Parents often describe feelings of guilt around not being able to tend to or parent their living children because of their grief. In some circumstances, parents can report feelings of resentment toward their living children for surviving when their other child did not. These sentiments, even if not openly expressed, are often sensed by surviving children and may result in complex grief experiences and identity crisis.

SIBLING EXPERIENCE
Spiritual Impact

Like their parents, siblings' spirituality is unique, because their beliefs are influenced by their own interpretations of what they have been taught and have observed from the media and world surrounding them. Their spirituality is further shaped by age, stage of psychosocial development and spiritual maturity.

James Fowler, head of the Center for Ethics in Public Policy and the Professions at Emory University, developed a theory of 6 stages of faith development, based on Erikson's theory of psychosocial development, which corresponds with developmental age.[14] His work has been instrumental in understanding how spirituality develops and has an impact on humans throughout life. These stages of faith are helpful in understanding how spirituality is understood and translated by children in their bereavement experiences. Fowler's categories applicable to children/adolescents include

- Stage 1—Intuitive-Projective faith (ages 3–7).[14] This stage picks up on Piaget's preoperational stage. Preschoolers tend to have a vivid imagination, in which anything is possible. They often have insights and intuitions particular to this age and may make associations to make sense of the world, which are also extrapolated to their conceptualization of their religion and/or god.[14]
- Stage 2—Mythic-Literal faith (school children but can be found also in adolescents and adults).[14] Children at the beginning of this stage tend to relate to myths and be concrete/literal. Trust tends to be a primary aspect of their relationship to God. Depending on their life experiences and phase of this stage, children may experience tension between mythic and literal understanding of God. This relationship can be particularly challenging when a child experiences illness and realize that their God is unable to heal them. This mythic conceptualization can also be challenged by their emerging development of logic.[14]
- Stage 3—Synthetic-Conventional faith (typically "has its rise and ascendancy in adolescence, but for many adults it becomes a permanent place of equilibrium").[14] It is typically during this period, either in adolescents or in early adulthood, that people begin to encompass greater ambiguity as well as acknowledge that people possess a diverse range of conceptualizations around

religious beliefs. A sense of belonging is crucial at this stage and, for some, community is more important than beliefs.[14]

In bereavement, the spiritual coping of siblings can also be affected by positive or negative spiritual beliefs or experiences. Children often relate positively that they continue to have a connection with a deceased sibling. They frequently share that their sibling is with God or in heaven and feel they can still talk to the sibling knowing that the brother or sister is watching over them. Such meaning-making narratives can be helpful in coping and processing as siblings move into adults.

In working with bereaved siblings, children should be encouraged to find ways to express their beliefs in a developmentally age-appropriate manner. Some children have clearly articulated ideas about their siblings and their spiritual beliefs about the death. Because all children may not express themselves in linear ways, engaging them through art and play can be effective ways in which to express spiritual and existential questions. Furthermore, experiences of negative religious beliefs may result in further anxiety and confusion. Similarly to adults, children may experience a crisis of faith following the death of loved one.

Recent research with cancer-bereaved siblings found that spiritual/religious coping (1 of 4 coping tools described) "was associated with sibling's experience of having worked through their grief two to nine years after the loss."[15] Research on spiritual beliefs and spiritual assessment with children is still in the infancy stage and there is need to develop more research in the subject of the bereavement of children as it relates to spirituality and the spiritual coping of children.

Emotional Processing/Behavioral Responses

Emotional processing and behavioral responses surrounding the death of a sibling can vary, depending on the psychosocial environment a child lives within as well as their personal stage of cognitive and emotional development. Not only do perceptions and reactions toward death vary among developmental stages but also the relationship with the death of a sibling can shift and change over time. Parent and caregiver responses to sensitive and vulnerable questions and behavioral needs of bereaved children can support both parental and familial bereavement.[16]

Questions that children may ask:

What's going to happen to them?
Am I going to die soon?
Did I do something wrong?
Why didn't the treatment work?
Will Mom and Dad be okay?
What is dying like? Will it hurt?
What happens after I die?
Is there anything I can do to bring my sibling back?

Important factors to assess when supporting a bereaved sibling are the micro, mezzo, and macro environments in which a child lives, respecting varied familial and cultural normative values.[17] There is a broad spectrum of what can be considered typical in regard to child development, with forms of attachment and cognitive norms shifting depending on the family the sibling is a part of, the community in which the sibling lives, and the supports the sibling may or may not have available.[17,18] Considering such a broad spectrum of typicality through a developmental lens could prove helpful when assessing the supportive needs of a bereaved child.

Developmental Understanding of End of Life and Grief

Infants and toddlers

From birth to approximately 2 years of age, infants and toddlers typically move through the sensorimotor stage of development, wherein object relations and attachment are navigated alongside physical and sensory exploration.[19,20] Babies do experience loss, primarily through their environment as they are learning object permanence.[21–23] Attachment is a central developmental theme within this stage, wherein inconsistency of environment and primary caregivers could lead to complicated feelings of attachment.[17,20–22] Children who experience stressors, such as trauma and loss, during this stage could exhibit behaviors, such as heightened sensitivity to unknown sounds, movements, or new people. They may become less engaged in distraction or play. When such a young child becomes a bereaved sibling, fostering opportunities for typical attachment can be helpful in creating a nurtured environment of development for both the child and the bereaved parent. Helpful interventions in supporting this population include supporting the use of transitional objects, nurturing a safe and connected familial environment, and therapeutic interventions for the bereaved parent so that they may be able to engage in such opportunities for typical development for their young child as they are able.[20,23]

Early childhood

Children who are between 2 years and 6 years of age are most typically moving through the preoperational stage of development, wherein ego development, incorporating new cognitive schema, and increased security in environmental exploration are prevalent.[18,19] From a cognitive standpoint, the concept of death may not be finite to young children within this stage. They may engage in magical thinking surrounding illness, hospitalization, and death, wherein unconnected actions or behaviors could be thought to effect the life of their sibling who has died.[16] Children within this stage may exhibit forms of regression in service of the ego, engaging in regressive behavior that reminds the child of a more familiar and safe developmental period. Such behaviors might include bed wetting, crawling, or using less formed language to express feeling.

These expressions of regression are not necessarily behavioral affects to be looked on as maladaptive but rather can be a child's way of learning how to incorporate new and vulnerable emotions during this expansive cognitive stage. Bereaved siblings within the preoperational period can benefit from play therapy as a way to work through and communicate about their experience and to integrate new schema of loss and death into their overall understanding of the world. Using play, drawing, and developmentally appropriate language, children can begin to express their perspectives of the experience of being a bereaved sibling while also providing opportunity to engage in their overall cognitive development.[24]

School-aged children

Children who are approximately the ages of 7 years to 12 yeras are within the concrete operational stage, wherein they are more solidified in their navigation of imaginative versus logical schemas of their environment.[18,19] They are beginning to explore their more social selves within peer relationships and have an ever-widening schema of emotional experience and understanding of the greater world.[18,19] During this stage, children tend to inhabit the understanding that death is a final cessation of life, although may believe death to happen only to those who are elderly or to animals and pets. Although they can use a clearer separation between life, illness, and death, it is a vulnerable realization to imagine that death can happen to children as well in the form of a sibling or loved one.[16]

To this end, children within this stage of development can benefit from developmentally appropriate play and story to communicate and work through the integration of new emotion and understanding. Children within this stage may ask more direct questions as they are able and can benefit from clear and open language surrounding death and dying.[24,25] Bereaved siblings within this and older developmental periods can benefit greatly from peer support groups or camps wherein bereaved children form connection and community. There may continue to be behaviors that serve as regression in service of protecting the ego, such as problems with sleeping alone at night and troubles concentrating at school. School counselors who are made aware of a bereaved sibling's experience and parent's utilization of supportive language surrounding this behavior can be beneficial in addressing the underlying emotional experience that might make such behaviors feel helpful to engage in for the child.

Adolescents and young adults

For the adolescent and young adult population within the formal operational stage, abstract thinking and integration of personal identity become central spheres of development that can be affected by the death of a sibling.[18,19] Cognitively, people who are ages 13 years to 18 years tend to understand that death is finite and could happen to anyone of any age. They are more able to comprehend the physical and biological process of illness and death, thus making their relationship with their sibling during the treatment and end-of-life process something that is often reflected on in bereavement.[16] In a bereaved sibling, grief can extend into loss of a sense of self and a feeling of isolation within identity and peer groups. Regressive behaviors can exhibit within this stage in the form of high-risk behaviors, engaging in activities that teens cognitively understand to possibly be of physical or emotional detriment to themselves.

Varied forms of support can aid parents and caregivers in supporting bereaved adolescents and young adults within this stage. Although still newly forming, teens may have internal ego strengths that can be used to build social connections, make personal meaning, or give name to their experience and inner emotional landscape surrounding the death of their sibling.[17] With respect to family systems and personal culture, young people within this stage of development can be capable of engaging in ritual and legacy building that could create space within which to build personal coping abilities alongside ongoing grief. Continued engagement in camps, online communities, or individualized therapeutic supports can prove beneficial while also recognizing that teens may additionally seek time alone or within their peer groups to find a sense of safety and security.

Providing opportunities for expression through multiple modalities can be useful for this population, particularly as they navigate the various stressors that any adolescent or young adult may experience. Tailoring outlets for ongoing grief to a person's interests and social needs could potentially aid parents in building a foundation for continued processing of grief into early adulthood.

Engaging Schools

When considering an ecological systems model, the crucial role of a school to a child during bereavement is apparent. Experiences there either positively or negatively have an impact on the remainder of the systems in their lives. Children spend much of their influential years in school and, therefore, engaging schools after the death of a sibling is imperative. Providers can relay to schools that the child and their death experience should not be treated as a stand-alone event but rather an experience encompassing child, peers, family, and school.[26]

By engaging schools and providing adequate staff training on helping children to navigate bereavement, providers can help to ensure that children's needs are addressed optimally. Through training, educators can become aware of the cognitive understanding of death at varying ages as well as the common behavioral, emotional, and psychological manifestations of childhood grief. After acquiring this understanding, teachers will be better able to recognize out of character behavior and address accordingly. Still, the school systems must remain aware of the teachers' need to process their own grief as well. These systems should put proactive and preventive responses enabling teachers to work through their grief to better support their students.[27–29]

If sufficiently equipped and adequately trained, teachers and school counselors can be trusted adults who are confident, knowledgeable of the school culture and typical peer interactions, and experts in using varying avenues of self-expression for children. Teachers and staff can provide a safe space for children to process their grief as well as work with children to create new rituals in memoriam of the deceased. As educators become aware of changes in behavior, they can relay these concerns to the parents/guardians of the child and refer the family to additional bereavement resources.

FAMILY RESOURCES/REFERRALS/COPING
Social Media

Families often reflect that feelings of isolation and estrangement from their social networks can be prohibitive in ongoing coping through grief. The sense of community that can be created through partaking in bereavement support groups led by trained facilitators can lead to reductions in such perceptions of isolation while providing both internal and external scaffolds of support. Several pediatric medical institutions have implemented such bereavement support groups, and the growing resources found virtually can additionally provide support for those who may find the outlet of social media connectivity and availability more suited to their lifestyle.

Support Groups

Such resources include the Healing Opportunities, Parent Exchanges (HOPE) bereavement support group, currently implemented at Boston Children's Hospital and Children's Hospital Los Angeles. The HOPE group is an 8-session closed group facilitated over the course of 16 weeks by trained chaplains, pediatric palliative care social workers, and nurse practitioners for bereaved parents whose children were served at these institutions. Online resources, such as Bereaved Parents of the USA, Healing Hearts for Bereaved Parents, and The Compassionate Friends provide educational tools, organized referrals for additional support, and virtual communities that can be used at the comfort and convenience of bereaved families.

Bereavement Camps

Family camps have additionally been shown to provide opportunity for therapeutic processing of a child's death as a greater family system while using developmentally appropriate outlets, such as play therapy and creative expression, to provide a foundation of support for ongoing bereavement. Such camps can provide group counseling based on age and relationship to the deceased child and artistic outlets for legacy building and creative expression as well as ongoing community support available outside of the camp setting. Camp Sunshine at Sebago Lake, Comfort Zone

Camp in California, and Camp Evergreen in Tennessee are among many such camps that provide tailored support for grieving parents and siblings.

Counseling and Psychotherapy

Individual and family counseling can also prove beneficial as a sole resource for bereaved families or in addition to the interventions outlined previously. Often, pediatric palliative care social workers provide initial bereavement follow-up after a child's death and can be helpful in referring families to local psychotherapists who can offer increased therapeutic support as needed.

Forgotten Grievers

The death of a child often has an impact on countless members of a family system and community system. The family system can include aunts, uncles, cousins, grandparents, and many others, depending on the structure of an individual family. Depending on the family system structure, relationship dynamics, culture of the family, and individual roles, a death likely has an impact on each family member in a unique manner. In considering pediatric death, it is crucial to recognize that how extended family members, such as grandparents, are grieving multiple losses simultaneously. For example, they likely grieve the loss of a grandchild while also grieving their own child's loss.

Other forgotten grievers may include members from additional communities in which the child interacted, such as faith systems or schools, as described previously. These forgotten grievers are prone to disenfranchised grief defined as grief that is not acknowledged by society.

PROVIDER EXPERIENCE
Personal Grief/Processing

An experience not often discussed among providers is the personal feelings of grief that may come when a patient dies. Although providers of all disciplines have varied encouragement in engaging with the experience that may be personally felt when caring for those who are at end of life, the nurturing of individual self-care can be of benefit in regards to tenability and viability within such work.[30–32]

Additionally, many hospitals facilitate regularly scheduled memorial services in an effort to provide opportunity for providers to acknowledge their patients' deaths. Furthermore, palliative care teams, spiritual care teams, and others may establish rituals to process death and emotional hardships together.

Palliative Care Role in Supporting Providers

As providers bear witness to the continual deaths of their patients and experience the compounded losses, they must find a certain balance between their apparent grief and their passion for the work they do each day. Staff distress can be described as the "emotional and psychological sensitivity that arises during these complex care experiences."[33]

Frequent opportunities for group and individual debriefings with a team social worker, chaplain, or psychologist may be beneficial. These spaces, whether formal or informal, can create a safe, nonjudgmental forum in which clinicians can bring their own hopes, worries, and challenges. When feeling supported and encouraged by colleagues, clinicians can reduce the potential risk factors for burnout, compassion fatigue, and vicarious traumatization.[16] Additionally, planning hospital memorial services can be a way for staff to honor and pay tribute to the patients who have died.

SUMMARY

The death of a child, no matter what the circumstances surrounding the death, often has an impact on various people within the family, health care team, and community. As providers, it is crucial to consider how to best support patients' families and also the various individuals impacted by this paradigm-shifting loss.

REFERENCES

1. Walsh F. A family resilience framework: innovative practice applications. Fam Relat 2002;51(2):130–7.
2. Bogensperger J, Lueger-Schuster B. Losing a child: finding meaning in bereavement. Eur J psychotraumatol 2014;5(1):22910.
3. Lowery M. Not just another day: families, grief and special days. Omaha (NE): A Center Corporation Resource; 1992.
4. Wolfelt A. Understanding your grief. Ten essential touchstones for finding hope and healing your heart. Fort Collins (CO): Companion Press; 2003.
5. Phelps AC, Lauderdale KE, Alcorn S, et al. Addressing spirituality within the care of patients at the end of life: perspectives of patients with advanced cancer, oncologists, and oncology nurses. J Clin Oncol 2012;30(20):2538–44.
6. Mako C, Galek K, Poppito SR. Spiritual pain among patients with advanced cancer in palliative care. J Palliat Med 2006;9(5):1106–13.
7. Marin DB, Sharma V, Sosunov E, et al. Relationship between chaplain visits and patient satisfaction. J Health Care Chaplain 2015;21:14–24.
8. Nash P, Parkes M, Hussain Z. Multifaith care for sick and dying children and their families, a multidisciplinary guide, 13. Philadelphia: Jessica Kingsley Publishers; 2015.
9. U.S. Public Becoming Less Religious, Modest drop in overall rates of belief and practice, but religiously affiliated americans are as observant as before. pew research center, religion & public life web site. 2015. Available at: http://www.pewforum.org/2015/11/03/u-s-public-becoming-less-religious/.htm. Accessed February 19, 2018.
10. Li J, Stroebe M, Chan CL, et al. Guilt in bereavement: a review and conceptual framework. Death Stud 2014;38(3):165–71.
11. Stroebe M, Stroebe W, Van De Schoot R, et al. Guilt in bereavement: the role of self-blame and regret in coping with loss. PLoS One 2014;9(5):e96606.
12. DeGroot JM, Carmack HJ. "It may not be pretty, but it's honest": examining parental grief on the caterpillar blog. Death Stud 2013;37(5):448–70.
13. Surkan PJ, Kreicbergs U, Valdimarsdóttir U, et al. Perceptions of inadequate health care and feelings of guilt in parents after the death of a child to a malignancy: a population-based long-term follow-up. J Palliat Med 2006;9(2):317–31.
14. Fowler J. Stages of faith, the psychology of human development and the quest for meaning. New York: Harper Collins Publishers; 1981. p. 133, 149, 172–3.
15. Lovgren M, Sween J, Steineck G, et al. Spirituality and religious coping are related to cancer-bereaved siblings' long term grief. Palliat Support Care 2017;1–5. https://doi.org/10.1017/S1478951517001146.
16. Wolfe J, Hinds P, Sourkes B. Textbook of interdisciplinary pediatric palliative care. Philadelphia: Elsevier Saunders; 2011.
17. Lesser JG, Pope DS. Human behavior and the social environment. Boston: Pearson Education Inc; 2011.
18. Donaldson M. Children's minds. New York: W.W. Norton & Company; 1978.

19. Piaget J. The origins of intelligence in children. London: Routledge and Kegan Paul; 1953.
20. Winnicott D. The use of an object. Int J Psychoanal 1969;20:711–6.
21. Brazelton TB, Cramer BG. The earliest relationship: parents, infants, and the drama of early attachment. Cambridge (England): Perseus Books; 1990.
22. Stern DN. The interpersonal world of the infant: a view from psychoanalysis and developmental psychology. New York: Basic Books; 1985.
23. Winnicott D. Transitional objects and transitional phenomena. Int J Psychoanal 1953;34:89–97.
24. Luby JL. Handbook of preschool mental health: development, disorders, and treatment. New York: The Guilford Press; 2006.
25. Brown S. Play: how it shapes the brain, opens the imagination, and invigorates the soul. New York: Penguin Group; 2009.
26. Reid J. School management and eco-systemic support for bereaved children and their teachers. International Journal of Children's Spirituality 2002;7(2): 193–207.
27. Black S. Research: how teachers and counselors can reach out to bereaved students. whenchildren grieve. Am Sch Board J 2005;192:28–30. Available at: http://www.asbj.com/.
28. Brown JA, Jimerson SR, Comerchero VA. Cognitive development considerations to support bereaved students: practical applications for school psychologists. Contemp Sch Psychol 2014. https://doi.org/10.1007/s40688-014-0018-6.
29. Swihart J, Silliman B, McNeil J. Death of a student: implications for secondary school counselors. The School Counselor 1992;40(1):55–60.
30. Back AL, Arnold RM, Tulsky JA, et al. On saying goodbye: acknowledging the end of the patient–physician relationship with patients who are near death. Ann Intern Med 2005;142(8):682–5.
31. Redinbaugh EM. Doctors emotional reactions to recent death of a patient: cross sectional study of hospital doctors. BMJ 2003;327(7408):185.
32. Rhodes-Kropf J, Carmody SS, Seltzer D, et al. "This is just too awful; i just can't believe i experienced that...": medical students' reactions to their "most memorable" patient death. Acad Med 2005;80(7):634–40.
33. Jonas DF, Bogetz JF. Identifying the deliberate prevention and intervention strategies of pediatric palliative care teams supporting providers during times of staff distress. J Palliat Med 2016;19(6):679–83.

The "Liaison" in Consultation-Liaison Psychiatry
Helping Medical Staff Cope with Pediatric Death

Anna C. Muriel, MD, MPH[a],*, Sarah Tarquini, PhD[a],
Sue E. Morris, PsyD[b]

KEYWORDS

- Consultation liaison • Bereavement • Burnout prevention • Pediatric death

KEY POINTS

- Pediatric consultation-liaison clinicians are well positioned to provide support, guidance, and systemic recommendations about how to help medical clinicians cope with the stresses of working with dying children.
- Interventions to support sustainability in this work need to occur at the institutional and team-based levels as well as in individual practice.
- Shared clinical work around challenging cases provides opportunities to engage with medical clinicians about their difficult experiences and provide reflection and support.
- Psychiatry services may also be in a role of advocating for institutionally based interventions that can help their medical colleagues.

INTRODUCTION

As child psychiatrists caring for youth with comorbid medical and psychiatric conditions, pediatric consultation-liaison (CL) psychiatrists are in the unique position of working closely with medical and nursing teams. The "consultation" may be to patients and families as well as to the primary medical teams. However, the "liaison" role, defined by Merriam-Webster as a "person who establishes and maintains communication for mutual understanding and cooperation," is specifically for the medical staff, with the ultimate goal of improving patient care. This liaison part of the job often involves support and psychological holding for the medical team

[a] Dana-Farber Cancer Institute, Boston Children's Hospital, Harvard Medical School, 450 Brookline Avenue, Boston, MA 02215, USA; [b] Department of Psychosocial Oncology and Palliative Care, Dana-Farber Cancer Institute, Boston Children's Hospital and Brigham and Women's Hospital, Harvard Medical School, 450 Brookline Avenue, Boston, MA 02215, USA
* Corresponding author.
E-mail address: amuriel@partners.org

Child Adolesc Psychiatric Clin N Am 27 (2018) 591–598
https://doi.org/10.1016/j.chc.2018.05.005   childpsych.theclinics.com

members as they care for patients. CL psychiatrists and their psychology and social work colleagues are sometimes embedded with subspecialty teams, such as oncology, transplant, complex care, intensive care, and palliative care, that regularly deal with dying children. Mental health providers may therefore be in the role of accompaniment, support, and guidance as these clinicians manage the emotional strain of watching their patients die. Although clinicians of other disciplines may serve these roles, this article specifically addresses the role of psychiatrists.

The loss of a loved person is one of the most intensely painful experiences any human being can suffer, and not only is it painful to experience, but also painful to witness, if only because we're so impotent to help.[1]

The compassionate care of the dying requires the ability to give of oneself without being destroyed in the process.[2]

Working with seriously ill patients can contribute to burnout in physicians and nurses throughout their training and practice over time. Burnout is a syndrome characterized by emotional exhaustion, cynicism and depersonalization, and feelings of ineffectiveness that may occur among people whose work is focused on serving others.[3] Medical clinicians who care for dying people may be particularly vulnerable to the emotional impact of patient deaths, which in turn may contribute to burnout. House staff, oncologists, palliative care doctors, and nurses and doctors working in intensive care units (ICUs) have been identified as having strong emotional responses to patient deaths that can affect patient care and physician well-being.[4–7]

The death of a child may be even more difficult for medical providers to cope with, because it may challenge beliefs about life and death and the way the world "should be," as well as one's professional effectiveness and capability. Most people in contemporary western societies hold a worldview that children will outlive their parents and that adults will live well into advanced years. When a child dies, these beliefs are thrown into question, and the greater the discrepancy between expectations and reality, the more difficult it can be to reconcile the death. Thus, the death of a child is considered to be one of the greatest losses a person can experience.[8,9] Medical providers may also acutely feel the suffering of parents and family members, contributing to the sense that the clinician failed in their charge to save the child's life. Pediatric ICU physicians have been shown to have burnout symptom rates of up to 70%,[10] and up to 86% of ICU nurses also report some symptoms.[11] Sudden child death[12] as well as protracted life-limiting illness such as cancer in children may be extremely stressful for clinicians and create a sense of helplessness. Pediatric oncologists have described feelings of sadness, exhaustion, self-questioning, guilt, and failure. These feelings may have impact outside of work, including irritability and disconnection from loved ones.[13] Physician burnout has been related to both decreased productivity and physician turnover,[14] and importantly, the quality of patient care.[15]

Learning to cope with the death of patients is an important skill that is often neglected in clinical training,[5,6,16,17] and yet needs to be cultivated throughout the course of a clinician's career.[4,7] Some clinicians find that working with seriously ill patients provides a meaningful perspective on life that allows them to appreciate things in a different way,[13] and personal characteristics, such as engagement and connection, may help clinicians be more resilient.[18] It is essential that clinicians gain insight into their own reactions to death and dying, bearing in mind they may hold a skewed view of the world given the pain and suffering they witness. Medical providers must reconcile their everyday work experience of illness and death, with human limitations for witnessing and absorbing the suffering of others, in order to sustain their work and thrive in their own lives.

SUPPORTING RESILIENCE IN MEDICAL PROVIDERS

Processing patient deaths is important to prevent burnout and compassion fatigue and requires that clinicians pay attention to self-care and developing coping strategies to tackle distressing emotions that inevitably arise in the care of very sick and dying children. Losses over time may accumulate, and if left unaddressed, have the potential to impact a clinician's personal and professional lives. Given that different patients will affect us in different ways at different stages in our lives, it is essential to put safeguards in place to help deal with grief and loss in a constructive manner. With prevention in mind, all clinicians should receive ongoing training to address the importance of self-care and how to incorporate these techniques into their daily lives at both work and home. At the same time, systems of care at the team and institutional levels must also provide opportunities for clinicians to minimize tasks that are draining and inefficient, and be able to focus on clinical practice that is effective and satisfying, including time to process patient deaths. There is still a limited evidence base for effective intervention to prevent or treat burnout, and both individual and workplace-based recommendations are being developed.[7] Nonetheless, CL clinicians are in a position to support their medical colleagues and implement systemic interventions that may be useful.

Case-Based Support

Vachon[2] states that "When caregivers begin to work in a setting where they will have regular exposure to dying persons, they should receive mentoring to help them deal with their grief in a manner that is, congruent with their personality and previous exposure to grief." CL psychiatrists and psychologists are well placed to facilitate such mentoring and recommend team practices that support resilience in the face of death. Sometimes support for medical and nursing colleagues comes in the consultation and accompaniment around particularly challenging cases. For example, when collaborating in the care of patients who have advancing disease, medical and nursing colleagues may express strong emotions or anticipatory grief; in that context, CL clinicians can provide a sounding board and reflective space for multidisciplinary colleagues. When seriously ill children also present with challenging psychiatric symptoms, such as persistent anxiety and depression, or parents have personality disorders that interfere with communication or medical decision making, the role of the CL clinician is essential. Medical physicians and nurses may feel even more helpless and ineffective as they struggle to manage these emotional and behavioral symptoms in addition to not being able to cure the underlying disease. When these complex patients die, medical providers may be left with complicated feelings of grief, guilt, and relief, that need to be processed and attenuated. Being familiar with the case and having worked alongside the multidisciplinary team allow the CL clinician to facilitate processing and debriefing soon after the death and share their own feelings and reflections about the case. Psychiatry clinicians must also attend to their own internal experience of the death and use appropriate individual self-care strategies.

Institutional Strategies

Institutions that care for sick and dying patients need a clear statement from senior management that endorses the importance of self-care for all staff, clinicians and administrative staff alike. Such a statement needs to be accompanied by regular, structured opportunities for clinicians to receive education, debriefing, and mentoring on an ongoing basis. Psychiatrists may be in a position to speak to these issues at the administrative level as health care leaders, or when called on to serve on institutional committees on clinical practice or patient safety and quality.

Institutional strategies include the following:

- Providing opportunities for staff to attend continuing education opportunities about end-of-life care and bereavement, ensuring reimbursement and protected time
  - Schwartz Rounds (http://www.theschwartzcenter.org/supporting-caregivers/schwartz-center-rounds/) is a specific opportunity for panel discussion and modeling of multidisciplinary management of difficult clinical situations and provides a safe space to process and share with the larger clinical community
  - Continuing education provides an opportunity for clinicians to explore and understand their reactions to death and to learn techniques to deal with distress or vicarious trauma that often accompanies caring for sick and dying patients
  - Discipline-specific education sessions support specific roles and skill development
  - Multidisciplinary educational opportunities help clinicians see different perspectives and how each discipline may support patients and families as well as each other, in unique ways
- Providing professional support for clinicians and staff through Employee Assistance Programs
- Holding annual institution or department memorial services for bereaved families and clinicians
  - Memorial services provide an opportunity for both bereaved families and clinicians and staff to come together to acknowledge the deaths of patients. Bereaved families not only find comfort in returning to the institution to honor their loved ones but also to have the opportunity to interact with team members who were involved in their loved one's care, and to say "goodbye" to the institution as whole. This is particularly important for those families who had a long relationship with the care team.

Team Strategies

Team-based strategies, promoted by the team leader, should be tailored to meet the specific needs of the team. Psychiatrists who are embedded in disease-based teams may be able to facilitate such interventions or provide guidance and support to team members who are creating them. These strategies may vary depending on the cause of death and the length of the relationship with the patient and family.

Team based strategies include the following:

- Debriefing opportunities, both formal and informal
  - Debriefing with the team creates a safe place where clinicians can express their thoughts and feelings about a certain case and process how they have been affected. From a psychological perspective, debriefing helps to normalize feelings and reduce isolation that some clinicians may feel, while at the same time, promoting communication and team cohesion. Formal debriefing is particularly helpful in situations involving sudden and unexpected death, and complex family or team dynamics because it provides a forum to review the details of events that occurred, ask questions, and express thoughts and feelings. Teams can identify what went well and where there were difficulties with a view to learning for future cases. Informal debriefing opportunities, such as an "open-door policy" with supervisors, checking in with a "buddy," or attending a peer support group, are other useful strategies.

- Memorial rituals or traditions that allow teams to acknowledge deceased patients in a systematic way
  - Memorial rituals can include annual team-only gatherings where deceased patients from the past year can be remembered and honored. This is a particularly helpful strategy for pediatric teams because it provides another level of sharing and opportunity for reflecting on the work they do.
  - "Bereavement rounds" can be incorporated into a team's regular clinical service. Ideally, they can be held during another scheduled team meeting, such as a staff or multidisciplinary team meeting. These types of rounds create a format for teams to remember patients who have recently died, discuss how their deaths impacted them personally or professionally, and identify those family members who might be "at-risk" of difficult bereavement outcomes, such as prolonged grief disorder, posttraumatic stress disorder, or other psychological or social difficulties. Early follow-up can be discussed and information passed to those clinicians responsible for providing bereavement outreach. Bereavement rounds also provide an opportunity for team members to sign sympathy cards.

Individual Strategies

CL clinicians may sometimes be pulled aside by a team member seeking guidance or support around their own complicated feelings about a case, or about more pervasive distress about their work with dying patients. Trainees or early career clinicians may need reassurance and reality testing about how hard it can be to deal with death, and how they are likely to be more impacted by deaths due to their inexperience. A sense of isolation with their emotional reactions about death is common among house staff[5] and can be relieved with support and providing context. More seasoned clinicians may also seek out consultation and support, and strong peer relationships and shared clinical experience can be a foundation for providing support, feedback, and recommendations to medical colleagues.

When clinicians think about self-care, they often focus on physical or social activities that occur outside work hours, such as exercise or spending times with friends. Although these activities are important in promoting well-being and maintaining a healthy perspective in life, we need to address self-care within the workplace, paying attention to how clinicians think about the work they do and the beliefs they hold. Promoting a culture within institutions where self-care is valued, and not seen as a sign of "weakness," is an important first step in helping staff to develop healthy attitudes and beliefs about the importance of self-care.

Realistic thinking about personal self-care includes the following:

- Self-care must be individualized and may evolve over time
- Adopt a "trial-and-error" approach to self-care strategies
- Incorporate strategies from the psychological, physical, and spiritual domains
- Establish an effective support system at work to complement support provided by external support systems
- Reach out for help if you feel out of your depth
- Develop ways to "actively grieve" for your patients[19]

Individual strategies following the death of a patient may include the following:

- Creating a pause during the workday
  - Spending time alone following a patient's death to reflect, pray, or cry can help clinicians acknowledge the death before moving on to the next patient.
- Challenging unhelpful or unrealistic thinking

○ How we think affects how we feel and how we behave. When a child dies, clinicians need to be able to identify unhelpful thoughts that can lead to negative emotional states (see more detailed information in later discussion on specific cognitive behavior therapy [CBT] strategies).

- Writing sympathy cards or making a condolence call
  ○ In addition to team cards, many clinicians find great benefit in writing a personal sympathy card and/or making condolence calls and may do so more the longer they practice.[17] This is particularly helpful when there has been a deep connection between the patient/family and the clinician. Writing a sympathy card or condolence note following the death of a child is a part of quality end-of-life care and an important self-care strategy. Not only do bereaved parents find comfort and support from receiving cards from the care team,[20] sending a sympathy card as a matter of routine practice can also help clinicians process their own feelings of grief and loss about their patients who die.
  ○ Suggestions for writing cards[21] include the following:
    ■ Express how you have been affected, for example, I was so sorry to hear of _____'s death.
    ■ Write something that reflects the patient's personality or the history you shared. Include stories about how their child touched your life or what you will remember.
    ■ If appropriate, emphasize the good job the parents did in caring for their child.
    ■ Adopt the motto, "Better late than never": it's always better to send a late card than not one at all. If some time has passed since the child's death, acknowledge the delay in sending the card, eg, *I am sorry that this card arrives late…* or *I only recently learned of ___'s death…*.
- Attending wakes and funerals
  ○ Many pediatric clinicians find attending wakes and funerals helpful in processing their grief because these traditions create a space away from the hospital for clinicians to remember their patients by paying their respects. Attending services with other team members creates a shared bereavement experience and fosters deeper collaboration. Families also find great comfort in seeing members of the care team. However, attendance at services is an individual decision for each clinician and should be respected either way. Institutional support to be away from work to attend services is also important.
- Providing bereavement follow-up
  ○ Providing bereavement follow-up to families or knowing that other team members are doing so can be a rewarding and healing conclusion to the relationship with the patient and family.[22] This follow-up might go beyond sending a sympathy card, to a phone call to check in on the family several weeks after the death, suggesting community resources, or inviting families back to the hospital for a follow-up meeting. Bereavement follow-up is an important component of quality end-of-life, for both families and clinicians.

A ROLE FOR COGNITIVE BEHAVIOR THERAPY

Drawing from psychology, many principles of CBT can be applied to self-care and how clinicians *think* about the work they do. These approaches may be woven into the strategies to help clinicians cope with death at all levels: institutional, team based, and individually. Although they may be most deeply implemented in individual debriefings and reflection, they may also be integrated in to clinician education, team discussions, or case-based learning.

The cognitive model proposes that dysfunctional thinking, which impacts an individual's mood and behavior, is common to all psychological disturbances.[23] When people learn to evaluate their thinking and develop more realistic and adaptive thinking patterns, they experience improvement in both their emotional state and their behavior. For lasting change, cognitive therapists work with their clients to examine deeply held cognitions, focusing on a person's beliefs about themselves, their world, and other people.

If, for example, following a child's death, the clinician thinks, *"this is terrible, we should have been able to save him—we let him down...,"* the clinician will most likely experience feelings of helplessness or a sense of failure. The clinician needs to learn to challenge his/her thinking. One question, based on CBT principles,[9] is *"how would I advise a colleague in the same situation?"* By answering this question, the clinician can generate a more realistic and helpful thought. For example, *"this is terribly sad, and even though I wish we could have saved him, we did everything possible given the circumstances..."*

The cognitive model lends itself to helping clinicians deal with the distress they experience related to patient care by offering a framework for identifying and challenging unhelpful thoughts and beliefs. Ideally, such training is introduced early in their careers to enable clinicians to develop a solid foundation of beliefs that are realistic and adaptive.

SUMMARY

Working with dying children has particular stresses for medical clinicians, and pediatric CL clinicians are well positioned to provide support, guidance, and systemic recommendations about how to help them cope and thrive. Interventions to support sustainability in the care of seriously ill children need to occur at the institutional and team-based levels as well as in individual practice. Clinical work around challenging cases provides opportunities to engage with medical clinicians about their difficult experiences and provide reflection and support. Psychiatry services may also be in a role of advocacy for institutionally based interventions that can help their medical colleagues.

REFERENCES

1. Bowlby J. Attachment and loss: loss, sadness, and depression, vol. III. New York: Basic Books; 1980.
2. Vachon MLS. Caring for the professional caregivers: before and after the death. In: Doka KJ, editor. Living with grief: before and after the death. Washington (DC): Hospice Foundation of America; 2007. p. 311–30.
3. Maslach C, Leiter MP. Understanding the burnout experience: recent research and its implications for psychiatry. World Psychiatry 2016;15(2):103–11.
4. Meier DE, Back AL, Morrison RS. The inner life of physicians and care of the seriously ill. JAMA 2001;286(23):3007–14.
5. Jackson VA, Sullivan AM, Gadmer NM, et al. "It was haunting...": physicians' descriptions of emotionally powerful patient deaths. Acad Med 2005;80(7): 648–56.
6. Sanchez-Reilly S, Morrison LJ, Carey E, et al. Caring for oneself to care for others: physicians and their self-care. J Support Oncol 2013;11(2):75–81.

7. Back AL, Steinhauser KE, Kamal AH, et al. Building resilience for palliative care clinicians: an approach to burnout prevention based on individual skills and workplace factors. J Pain Symptom Manage 2016;52(2):284–91.

8. Williams J. Pediatric death: a focus on health care providers. Arch Pediatr Adolesc Med 2010;164(4):311–3.

9. Morris SE. Overcoming grief: a self-help guide using cognitive behavioral techniques. London: Constable Robinson; 2008.

10. Garcia TT, Garcia PC, Melon ME, et al. Prevalence of burnout in pediatric intensivists: an observational comparison with general pediatricians. Pediatr Crit Care Med 2014;15(8):e347–53.

11. Moss M, Good VS, Gozal D, et al. An official critical care societies collaborative statement-burnout syndrome in critical care health-care professionals: a call for action. Chest 2016;150(1):17–26.

12. Truog RD, Christ G, Browning DM, et al. Sudden traumatic death in children: "we did everything, but your child didn't survive". JAMA 2006;295(22):2646–54.

13. Granek L, Bartels U, Scheinemann K, et al. Grief reactions and impact of patient death on pediatric oncologists. Pediatr Blood Cancer 2015;62(1):134–42.

14. Dewa CS, Loong D, Bonato S, et al. How does burnout affect physician productivity? A systematic literature review. BMC Health Serv Res 2014;14:325.

15. Dewa CS, Loong D, Bonato S, et al. The relationship between physician burnout and quality of healthcare in terms of safety and acceptability: a systematic review. BMJ Open 2017;7(6):e015141.

16. Hough CL, Hudson LD, Salud A, et al. Death rounds: end-of-life discussions among medical residents in the intensive care unit. J Crit Care 2005;20(1):20–5.

17. Merel SE, Stafford MM, White AA, et al. Providers' beliefs about expressing condolences to the family of a deceased patient: a qualitative and quantitative analysis. J Palliat Med 2015;18(3):217–24.

18. Kearney MK, Weininger RB, Vachon ML, et al. Self-care of physicians caring for patients at the end of life: "Being connected... a key to my survival". JAMA 2009; 301(11):1155–64. E1151.

19. Worden JW. Grief counseling and grief therapy: a handbook for the mental health practitioner. 2nd edition. New York: Springer Publishing Company; 1991.

20. Donovan LA, Wakefield CE, Russell V, et al. Hospital-based bereavement services following the death of a child: a mixed study review. Palliat Med 2015; 29(3):193–210.

21. Morris SE, Block SD. Grief and bereavement. In: Grassi L, Riba M, editors. Clinical psycho-oncology:an international perspective. West Sussex (England): Wiley-Blackwell; 2012. p. 271–80.

22. Milberg A, Appelquist G, Hagelin E, et al. "A rewarding conclusion of the relationship": staff members' perspectives on providing bereavement follow-up. Support Care Cancer 2011;19(1):37–48.

23. Beck J. Cognitive behavior therapy: basics and beyond. New York: The Guilford Press; 2011.

Social Media Consequences of Pediatric Death

David Buxton, MD[a],*, Taylor R. Vest, MSW[b]

KEYWORDS

- Social media • Pediatrics • Bereavement • Adolescent • Legacy • Deceased • Grief
- Teenagers

KEY POINTS

- Most teenagers have a "social media portfolio" and use many social media platforms.
- Social media is changing the landscape of grief and bereavement in adolescents and adults.
- Social media can be a tool to allow youth to stay connected with previous friends but also an opportunity to engage with other individuals facing similar challenges.
- This use of the Internet social networks to express feelings of grief may be a positive outlet for teens who are grieving.

INTRODUCTION TO SOCIAL MEDIA

Social media is ubiquitous in our current society. It is an intense force that has become a vital tool for social engagement of children and teenagers. To have a relationship with another peer includes connecting through multiple digital affiliations, including Facebook, Instagram, YouTube, and Snapchat. Child and adolescent psychiatrists will need to be more familiar with social networking, as it plays a vital element of a teenager's inner and external worlds.

The American Academy of Child and Adolescent Psychiatry Facts for Families in 2011 lists a series of benefits that include staying connected with friends, developing new social contacts with similar interests, sharing content of self-expression such as art work/music, and assisting in development of an identity.[1] Unfortunately, social networking also has created new challenges and struggles for adolescents to navigate. One example of this is "virtual bullying," in which peers share negative content or embarrassing information on social media. These posts can go viral, so instead of just a one group bully it can spread to the entire school. Many of these cases are

Disclosure Statement: Dr D.C. Buxton reports Leadership Fellowship Committee Member, American Psychiatric Association; Fellowship Committee Member, American Psychoanalytic Association; American Lead, The Digital Legacy Association.
[a] Center for Palliative Psychiatry, 3101 Kensington Avenue, Unit 403, Richmond, VA 23221, USA; [b] Virginia Commonwealth University, Richmond, VA, USA
* Corresponding author.
E-mail address: dbuxton@palliativepsychiatry.com

connected to impulsive decision making in which a teen shares too much information or inappropriate photos/videos.

Previously, children were exposed to traditional media (television, radio, periodicals) that were externally created by production companies with limitations around material content. Unlike traditional media, social media is not just consumed by users, but teenagers are creating the active content. The boundaries between what is appropriate or inappropriate is not defined by outside forces, and information is constantly flowing back and forth. Furthermore, youth are engaging[2] with digital content as young as 4 months compared with children in 1970 who began television screening at age 4 years old. A trend has begun to show less engagement with traditional media and an uptick in social media use. The Kaiser Family Foundation reported that in 2011, 52% of children 0 to 8 years of age had access to a mobile device, and by 2013 it had increased to 75%.[3] Currently, 3 of 4 teenagers own a phone and up to 50% have reported feeling "addicted to it."[2]

Recent Pew reports have demonstrated that most 13-year-old to 17-year-old teenagers have a "social media portfolio" in which they use multiple platforms to connect. The rates of site use are Facebook (71%), Instagram (52%), Snapchat (41%), and (Twitter 33%). As most teenagers engage with Facebook, further details show that typical teenagers have approximately 145 friends with equal use between boys and girls.[4] In addition, data have shown teenagers spend approximately 1 hour and 11 minutes a day, 7 days a week on social media.[5]

Research has begun to expand on increasing the understanding and effects of social media. Well-known psychological mechanisms are now seen in a digital form, such as social comparison (comparing oneself to others, either better or worse), impression management (highlighting attractive elements of themselves or life while withholding negative aspects), and self-disclosure (revealing confidential information about themselves). By having another venue to use these methods, social media can help with developmental tasks of autonomy, intimacy, and peer engagement. Most teenagers report that social media is a positive experience, with an increase in self-esteem, a safe place for self-exploration, and an increase in social capital (access points for social relationships). Research has also shown negative consequences with associations of an increase in depression, social anxiety, exposure to inappropriate content, and cyberbullying.[5]

SOCIAL MEDIA AND LIFE-LIMITING ILLNESSES

A life-limiting illness can be a traumatic experience and forces an individual to confront his or her own mortality. This can lead to a wide range of psychosocial challenges and a feeling of isolation. For adolescents who are working through the developmental task of learning how to have relationships outside of their family, a larger deficit may occur. Social media can be a tool to allow youth to stay connected with previous friends but also an opportunity to engage with other individuals facing similar challenges.[6] The ability to connect with peers, such as those with cancer, via social media has led to online de facto community support groups. An immense power can be derived from the ability to connect 24 hours a day/7 days a week anywhere in the world with a virtual friend facing similar obstacles.[7] For individuals who have rare disorders or are isolated by geographic locations, social media opens a possibility to find other individuals with their disease without leaving home.[8] Teenagers have been reported to dialogue about complications from their disease, such as fertility, relationships, loss of autonomy, interruptions in school/work, and financial implications, through social media.[9]

Another novel event that has arisen from these social networks is the use of "crowd-sourcing" (obtaining information from an evolving online community) treatment options and alternatives to assist in making more informed decisions. Some health care professionals are concerned about misinformation through this avenue, with one study pointing out that 19% of cancer information shared on Facebook was inaccurate.[10]

Social media also can be helpful for caregivers/parents as an outlet for communication. For example, review of parents who have a child with cancer use social media demonstrates theme of a desire to share cancer journey, sharing emotional stress, advocacy about pediatric cancer, fundraising, and requesting support.[11]

DIGITAL LEGACY

It has been hypothesized that most individuals will be remembered for approximately 70 years based on the fact that many people cannot name their great-grandparents. For emperors, kings, and other royals, a significant amount of energy and wealth was devoted to trying to create ongoing legacies to avoid being lost to history. Social media has democratized this process through providing an ongoing account of thoughts, pictures, and videos that theoretically can live on forever via a digital legacy.[12] Most users have thought very little of this concept, with close to 90% of individuals making no plans for their accounts.[13] Some companies, like DeadSocial, have begun to enter this space through digital end-of-life planning and now offer the ability to pre-program a future postmortem post to friends and family through Facebook and Twitter for a later date, that is, birthdays, anniversaries, and so on.[12] Currently, there is no set industry norm for how companies are dealing with death and digital legacies. See **Table 1** for policies.

As this concept can sound strange to digital immigrants, teenagers who are digital natives are more integrated with their technology and social media. A good example of an adolescent who used social media and created a digital legacy was Ben Breedlove. Ben was diagnosed with hypertrophic cardiomyopathy at an early age. He underwent multiple surgeries, including implantation of a pacemaker. In his early teens, Ben became very active on YouTube creating his own channels in which he provided

Table 1		
Social media policies after the death of a member		
Platform	**Procedure**	**Abilities**
Facebook	Legacy Contact	• Write a post that will remain at the top of a profile • Update a profile photo • Respond to friend requests • Cannot read private messages • Account also can be deleted
Instagram	Verified next-of-kin can have account memorialized or deleted	None
Twitter	Verified immediate family member of the deceased can delete account	None
LinkedIn	Verified next-of-kin can have an account deleted	None
Snapchat	Verified next-of-kin can have account deleted	None
Tumblr	Verified next-of-kin can have account deleted	None

relationship and love advice to peers. On December 18, 2011, Ben posted a 2-part video called "This is my life" in which he shared his experience living with a life-limiting illness and 3 near-death experiences through the use of prewritten note cards. One week later, on Christmas Eve at the age of 18, Ben died from a heart attack. His family did not find his video until the day after his death. The video went viral with most major traditional media across the world covering his story and thousands of teen-agers across the country responding via social media.[14] Currently, "This is my life" had been viewed by more than 9 million people on YouTube with more than 15,000 comments.[15]

DIGITAL BEREAVEMENT

Bereavement refers to the phase of mourning and grief following the death of a beloved person. Mourning is the term used to portray the public formalities or symbols of bereavement, such as holding funeral services or wearing black clothing. In the past, mourning was most commonly experienced in isolation. Because of the growing nature of digital bereavement, "grief shared, is grief relieved" tends to be a more commonly held belief today.[16] Thanatechnology was coined by researcher Carla Sofka to describe the way people use the Internet to display their feelings of grief when a loved one has died. This use of the Internet social networks to express feelings of grief may be a positive outlet for teens who are grieving.[16] Similar to how people use Facebook to commemorate life events, people also use Facebook to memorialize those who have died. Social media is allowing people a new outlet to express their grief.

For many adolescents, suddenly losing a peer forces them face their own immor-tality. A study of 100 college undergraduate students found that social network sites like Facebook are changing the landscape of how teens mourn.[17] On discovering that someone had died, 45% of students in this study disclosed to immediately visiting the Facebook page of the deceased. Fourteen percent of the students reported changing their profile picture to that of the deceased or to a picture of a ribbon honoring the deceased. Actions such as posting on the deceased person's wall, almost as if teens were maintaining a relationship with the deceased as a way to cope with their loss, and often posting to the deceased as if the deceased could read the posts were popular with respondents of this study.

Facebook has more than 30 million deceased users with active profile pages. Aside from deleting contact information, deceased individuals' profile pages stay intact. Facebook users can designate a "legacy contact" control over the profile to make mi-nor changes or add new connections post-death who would like to join in the grieving process. A content analysis of 2533 messages posted on 10 deceased individuals' Facebook profile pages disclosed that messages to the deceased reflect 3 themes: Processing the Death, Remembering the Deceased, and Continuing the Connection.[18] A message analysis revealed that public posts relating to processing the death and reminiscing the deceased peak directly after loss and then declined in frequency, whereas private messages indicating prolonged connections increase with time.

Virtual memorials, or Web cemeteries, are defined as online spaces that provide a place to honor and remember the deceased, including memorial Web pages, online funeral home guest books, blogs, discussion boards, and social networking sites. Four major characteristics of online memorials that distinguish them from offline for-mats are flexible timing, access, visiting, and sharing. Virtual memorials allow for flex-ible timing, permitting the bereaved to access the memorial at their own convenience. This feature allows users to mourn and grieve at any time. The user's access to the virtual memorials is unrestricted, allowing any user the ability to participate despite geographic location. Users are able to share with others who wish participate in the remembrance of the deceased. Connecting through a virtual memorial has potential to act as a healing mechanism for the bereaved, as it often enables the mourner express what is difficult to say to others.[18]

Online obituaries, such as Legacy.com, are evolving and provide a space for the bereaved to express grief. These online obituaries can vary widely in form and context. Mourners who visit these sites included the deceased family, friends, colleagues, and even strangers. One study examined obituaries linked to online guest books of major US daily newspapers and categorized mourners' behaviors into 3 categories: sending messages to the deceased and the deceased's family, expressing emotions, and telling stories.[19] Mourner posts were also categorized into 2 grieving functions: sense-making (how the grieving makes sense of the death, through expressions of shock, spirituality, lamentations, questions, and prose) and continuing bonds (how the grieving renegotiates a new identity with the deceased, through posting emotions and memories).[20]

The thought that people should move forward after death frequently permeates contemporary culture and restricts the ability for the bereaved to process their loss and what life will be like without the deceased. Past models of grief communication consider the end goal of the grieving process to be closure and acceptance, a breaking of connections with the deceased so that the bereaved can move on with their life. Social media and virtual memorials have allowed for continuing ties and a restructuring of the processes of grief and bereavement. Instead of severing ties with the deceased, there is now space for a renegotiation of the relationship between the deceased and bereaved in a way that can become a normal and necessary part of the grieving process. This restructuring does not mean the severing of ties, but rather becomes a redefining of the bond and what it means to the bereaved. Despite many fearing grieving publically, many people found comfort in the deceased's Facebook profile page and discovered it common to express their grief and maintain the restructured relationship with the deceased.[21]

Because of the public nature of Facebook communication, people who did not personally know the deceased, known as emotional rubberneckers, can find virtual memorial groups and observe people grieve the loss of their friend or family member. Rubbernecking seems to be a way by which people who did not know the deceased coped with a death that affected them in some way. A subset of rubberneckers likely includes lurkers, or individuals who view the virtual memorial groups and public dialogue without participating in writing messages. In some cases, lurkers may only observe to get a better perspective of grief, without the pressure to contribute in the conversation. Most Facebook rubberneckers seemed to have positive objectives for viewing in the online memorial groups. Rubbernecking can be a beneficial and constructive endeavor for those responding to the death.[22]

SUMMARY

Social media is an important part of teenagers' lives and allows them to connect in ways that no previous generation has ever faced. The creation and maintenance of these affiliations is interwoven into their peer relationships as one way to foster deeper connections and avoid isolation. For those adolescents who are faced with life-limiting illnesses, social media opportunities allow them to remain active in previous relationships while also fostering new ties with similarly sick teens. When working with this population, providers need to be aware of the concept of digital legacy, as it can not only affect the patient but his or her "real" and digital peers. In addition, providers should be familiar with how this new generation uses social media as part of their bereavement.

REFERENCES

1. Facts for families, children, and social networking. Aacap.org. 2018. Available at: http://www.aacap.org/App_Themes/AACAP/docs/facts_for_families/100_children_and_social_networking.pdf. Accessed January 22, 2018.
2. Chassiakos Y, Radesky J, Christakis D, et al. Children and adolescents and digital media. Pediatrics 2016;138(5):e20162593.
3. Rideout V. Zero to eight: children's media use in America. San Francisco (CA): Common Sense Media; 2011.
4. Lenhart A. Teens, technology and friendships. PEW Research Center: Internet, science & tech. 2018. Available at: http://www.pewinternet.org/2015/08/06/teens-technology-and-friendships/. Accessed January 27, 2018.
5. Uhls Y, Ellison N, Subrahmanyam K. Benefits and costs of social media in adolescence. Pediatrics 2017;140(Supplement 2):S67–70.
6. Gibson F, Hibbins S, Grew T, et al. How young people describe the impact of living with and beyond a cancer diagnosis: feasibility of using social media as a research method. Psychooncology 2016;25(11):1317–23.
7. Myrick J, Holton A, Himelboim I, et al. #Stupidcancer: exploring a typology of social support and the role of emotional expression in a social media community. Health Commun 2015;31(5):596–605.
8. Primack B, Shensa A, Sidani J, et al. Social media use and perceived social isolation among young adults in the US. Am J Prev Med 2017;53(1):1–8.
9. Perales M, Drake E, Pemmaraju N, et al. Social media and the adolescent and young adult (AYA) patient with cancer. Curr Hematol Malig Rep 2016;11(6):449–55.
10. Gage-Bouchard E, LaValley S, Warunek M, et al. Is cancer information exchanged on social media scientifically accurate? J Cancer Educ 2017. [Epub ahead of print].
11. Gage-Bouchard E, LaValley S, Mollica M, et al. Cancer communication on social media. Cancer Nurs 2017;40(4):332–8.
12. Taubert M, Watts G, Boland J, et al. Palliative social media. BMJ Support Palliat Care 2014;4(1):13–8.
13. What is a digital legacy? The digital legacy association. The digital legacy association. 2018. Available at: https://digitallegacyassociation.org/about/what-is-a-digital-legacy/. Accessed January 25, 2018.
14. Ben Breedlove. Enwikipediaorg. 2018. Available at: https://en.wikipedia.org/wiki/Ben_Breedlove. Accessed January 22, 2018.
15. Ben Breedlove This is my story - (Part 1 and 2). YouTube. 2011. Available at: https://www.youtube.com/watch?v=dUUjNFbL3XU. Accessed January 24, 2018.
16. Goldschmidt K. Thanatechnology: eternal digital life after death. J Pediatr Nurs 2013;28(3):302–4.
17. Carroll B, Landry K. Logging on and letting out: using online social networks to grieve and to mourn. Bull Sci Technol Soc 2010;30(5):341–9.
18. Bouc A, Han S, Pennington N. "Why are they commenting on his page?": using Facebook profile pages to continue connections with the deceased. Comput Human Behav 2016;62:635–43.

19. Hume J, Bressers B. Obituaries online: new connections with the living—and the dead. Omega (Westport) 2009-2010;60(3):255–71.
20. McCartney P. Online obituaries and memorials. MCN Am J Maternal Child Nurs 2014;39(3):206.
21. Pennington N. You don't de-friend the dead: an analysis of grief communication by college students through Facebook profiles. Death Stud 2013;37(7):617–35.
22. DeGroot J. "For whom the bell tolls": emotional rubbernecking in Facebook memorial groups. Death Stud 2013;38(2):79–84.

Assisting the School in Responding to a Suicide Death: What Every Psychiatrist Should Know

Emily J. Aron, MD[a,*], Jeff Q. Bostic, MD, EdD[a],
Julie Goldstein Grumet, PhD[b], Sansea Jacobson, MD[c]

KEYWORDS

- School-based mental health • Suicide • Postvention • Suicide contagion

KEY POINTS

- Suicide among school-age children has significant effects on the student population.
- Evidence-based suicide postvention guidelines are available to help guide schools following a student suicide.
- Child psychiatrists and mental health clinicians can play a variety of roles in the postvention process and can aid schools in a variety of ways through a well-thought-out response (ie, understanding grief reactions based on developmental levels, creating a crisis response team, advising schools on how to speak with the media).
- Providing suicide postvention following a student suicide is also a part of suicide prevention programming in schools.

Suicide is the second leading cause of death among young people between the ages of 15 and 19.[1] In 2016, 2439 children between the ages of 13 and 19 died by suicide,[2] and approximately 8% of high school students report making suicide attempts each year.[3] Additional concerns involve those students who are bereaved following a student suicide. Andriessen and colleagues[4] reported that past year prevalence of exposure to suicide among adolescents was approximately 4% and lifetime prevalence was approximately 21% (with suicide being more likely by a peer than a family member). The number of people impacted by each suicide ranges from 10 to 147, with 1 in 5 reporting devastating effects or major life disruption[5]; moreover, exposure to a

Disclosure Statement: None.
[a] Department of Psychiatry, Medstar Georgetown University Hospital, 2115 Wisconsin Avenue Northwest, Washington, DC 20007, USA; [b] Suicide Prevention Resource Center, Education Development Center, Inc, 1025 Thomas Jefferson Street, Suite 700West, Washington, DC 20007 43, USA; [c] Department of Psychiatry, Western Psychiatric Institute & Clinic, UPMC, 3811 O'Hara Street, E503, Pittsburgh, PA 15213, USA
* Corresponding author.
E-mail addresses: emily.j.aron@gunet.georgetown.edu; emilyaron@gmail.com

Child Adolesc Psychiatric Clin N Am 27 (2018) 607–619
https://doi.org/10.1016/j.chc.2018.05.007
1056-4993/18/© 2018 Elsevier Inc. All rights reserved.

suicide increases vulnerability to mental health issues, such as depression[6] and risk of suicide.[7]

A school is well positioned to provide support for students in the aftermath of a suicide. First, schools provide a familiar environment where students can continue to learn and thrive amid routines and people they know well. Second, school-based clinicians can provide mental health screening and targeted support to vulnerable youth to contain additional adverse outcomes, including the rare, but potentially lethal phenomenon of suicide contagion. Third, by promoting psychoeducation and open dialogues, schools can combat the stigma and shame that too often surround mental illness and suicide. Fourth, schools can offer frequent contact with individuals who are struggling with common trauma-related reactions (eg, ruminating on a "missed" opportunity to avert the suicide, feeling unsure how to respond, or feeling guilty for moving forward after a suicide). Finally, schools also have the unique opportunity to help scaffold the community (both school and town/city) to promote a wider healing after the tragedy of a school suicide.

Typically, a response to a student suicide is handled by the school mental health staff available in the local school district. However, the school may also consider reaching out to local child psychiatrists who can meaningfully and uniquely contribute to the healing process. Child psychiatrists may be contacted to assist with the initial crisis response, provide day-to-day guidance in the weeks after the death, and/or to gauge long-term progress. Having access to available resources and understanding the "dos and don'ts" of how to respond to a student suicide eases the navigation of an innately challenging situation. As champions of health and well-being for youth, child psychiatrists can serve as advocates for their communities to advance suicide prevention and promote healthier schools.

Having a coordinated plan to help students in the aftermath of suicide will lead to a faster recovery and return to precrisis academic and emotional functioning. When schools are not able to implement a postvention plan, there is risk for increase in psychological difficulties, disciplinary referrals, absences, and subsequently, a negative impact on the learning environment.[8] Emerging evidence provides clarity for specific steps to take during the immediate days, weeks, and months after a student suicide. There are a variety of online resources that schools might find helpful, including state-specific suicide prevention plans at the Suicide Prevention Resource Center (SPRC) Web site (http://www.sprc.org/states) and Substance Abuse and Mental Health Services Administration's Preventing Suicide: A Toolkit for High Schools, which provide an excellent starting place for developing a comprehensive approach to suicide prevention as well as response to a student suicide. Using these resources and examining the literature, what follows is a guide highlighting the elements of the school response to student suicide intersecting with the role of the child psychiatrist.

RESPONDING TO A SCHOOL SUICIDE: A TIMELINE

Postvention is the term used to describe the interventions implemented following a school crisis. More specifically, the term suicide postvention is defined as "activities developed by, with or for suicide survivors in order to facilitate recovery after suicide and to prevent adverse outcomes including suicidal behavior."[9] Recommendations encompass both the procedures of responding to a suicide and the mental health interventions that are warranted and invaluable in the days to months that follow. Just as grief unfolds over time, it is natural for a school community to experience an evolving process after the tragic loss of a student. As such, conceptualizing a school response via a chronologic timeline is helpful in providing a roadmap and also detailing a staged response that will parallel the grieving process of students and the larger school community.

Typically, school responses to a suicide occur in 3 stages:

1. Immediately following a suicide: this interval usually consists of the immediate messaging to the school community, initial student/staff reactions, and funeral/service participation; usually, this phase lasts about 1 week after the school learns of the suicide;
2. Student reequilibration: this is the interval when most students return to regular functioning, while other students may struggle or even deteriorate, and thus require more intervention support. This is also the interval during which the school community begins moving forward with the legacy/memory of the student; this usually lasts for weeks to months;
3. School reequilibration: the long-term aftermath of the suicide includes integration of the suicide into school events, such as graduation or the anniversary of the event. Another important component of this period is the implementation of systematic changes, often with improved screening, new or altered service provisions, and sustainable program changes to address risk factors (eg, substance abuse, bullying).

Stage 1: Immediate Suicide Postvention (up to 1 Week After Suicide)

There are several resources that provide different steps that schools can take immediately following a student suicide death. The child psychiatrist can assist the school's crisis response team in implementing these steps. Each step encompasses a need for an in-depth understanding of the mental health needs of various groups (family of deceased, school staff, parents in the community, students).

The items listed are some of the key steps that schools should take. Each circumstance is unique, so it is best to address these items in an order that makes sense for the specific situation:

- Verify the student's death with the family when possible. Social media lends itself to the distribution of misinformation; therefore, verifying that information is accurate is necessary.
- Communicate condolences to the family and assist with a message to provide the school community that is consistent with the family's wishes.
- Have the school's crisis team meet (preferably before students arrive to school) to identify responsibilities:
  ○ Identify students likely to be impacted by this event and who will reach out to those students.
  ○ Determine who will provide information to parents/community, and the school's response, regarding this event.
- Notify and then assemble the school staff to share facts about the event and funeral details, and anticipate student questions. It is not necessary to go into detail about how the student died, but all staff and the crisis team should have a clear, factually correct narrative based on the events that occurred as well as what the family wants shared. School staff also benefits from crisis intervention themselves with ample opportunity to discuss reaction to the suicide death of a student.
- Clarify the process (the when and where information) to notify students.
- Prepare school staff with the following:
  ○ What to say to students about this event
  ○ How students can express condolences to the family (and "remember" the student)

○ Provide information about depression, suicide, hotlines, availability of counselors, feelings that often emerge after a death, and so forth as is age appropriate for their students
- Provide ongoing Crisis Team Check-In throughout the day to clarify impacts and needs.
  ○ Are outside providers needed to speak with student/staff groups?
- School staff should debrief at the end of the day to discuss issues that emerged, students that might need additional support, and plan to address.

Notifying the staff and students

After working with the bereaved family to determine how and what information is to be shared, the focus then shifts to disseminating information to the school personnel and students. Staff should be notified about the death before students are formally told. Ideally, staff can be brought together to hear of the student's death and to ask any questions. At this time, a prepared statement to be read to students is shared with staff to allow for any modifications or revisions before the information is shared with students. It also provides an opportunity for school staff to get more information on what to share, how to respond to students' questions, where to direct them for help, how to recognize students who might need some additional support, and common student reactions to grief.

Initial information about the death is often shocking and can invoke intense feelings (from sadness to anger to shutting down) and thus should be addressed with students in small groups (eg, in their homeroom). It is important *not* to communicate the death through "public address system announcements" or large meetings. For students who are distraught, having an identified place (and counseling staff) to meet, in addition to the initial classroom announcement and discussion, can help students process their reactions.

Notification of the death to parents/community

Working with natural supports (ie, parents, coaches and other adults in the community who interact with students) can help foster an air of care and understanding. Parents also experience intense emotional reactions, and some will be at a loss of how to best help their children. The child psychiatrist can help schools prepare, if asked, a statement, but also help anticipate reactions of parents and how students may be affected by witnessing adults in distress. Schools can help shore up support for their students by reaching out to parents via letters and parent meetings about what occurred, how the school is managing it, and what resources exist. In-person meetings can both alleviate community concerns and enlist parental support in reaching vulnerable youth. A child psychiatrist or other mental health professional may be asked to be present at one of these meetings on topics, such as typical youth responses to a sudden death, symptoms of adolescent depression, risk factors and behaviors that indicate concern, and available resources. Because large meetings can be unwieldy and lead to scapegoating and blaming, it is recommended that the school divide the initial parent meeting into 2 parts. The first part reviews the facts related to the student death (respecting the family's wishes and preferably after reviewing the message with parents directly) and dissemination of general information about the school's response without opening the meeting up to discussion. The second part of the meeting should divide the parents into small group discussions with trained crisis counselors on site to answer questions and provide support. A sample agenda for a parent meeting is available in After a Suicide: A Toolkit for Schools.[10]

Interaction with local media

Designating an identified crisis team member (usually the Principal) to interact with the media and channeling all media personnel to that person is most helpful to provide consistent messages. Staff benefit from knowing to route all media contacts/requests to this person and media interviews of students on school grounds may make the school feel less safe; similarly, media participation at parent/student/staff meetings may allow sensitive information to be taken out of context and then broadcast repeatedly, often unhelpfully, which can impede community healing.

Ideally, the school spokesperson should prepare a written statement for release to the media. The statement should not provide details of the death itself. Although it may include condolences to the survivors of the deceased, the focus should be on describing the positive postvention efforts designed to help student survivors as well as practical information about mental health and community resources available for struggling youth. The school should provide local media with Recommendations for Reporting on Suicide, available at http://reportingonsuicide.org/wp-content/themes/ros2015/assets/images/Recommendations-eng.pdf.[11]

School staff discussion with students

Staff will likely have several moments, both immediately and over subsequent weeks to months, when the topic of suicide will be brought up by students. **Table 1** provides ways that staff can talk about issues that may come up following a student suicide.

Student and staff reactions to the suicide

Each survivor experiences the loss differently, often with unanticipated emotions overwhelming their rational understanding of death. Moreover, although the suicide may involve a high school student, the siblings, classmates, friends, and community members impacted will cross all ages and developmental levels.

Although there is a common set of initial responses, including shock, sadness, anger, and disbelief, it is important to help the community understand that there is no correct way to grieve, and that each person may grieve on a different timeline (ie, the school will need to be flexible because various students and staff go through this initial grieving process at different paces). When feasible, it is preferable to continue school, classes, or scheduled activities, because the day-to-day structure of the regular school routine can provide comfort to the student community (extenuating circumstances do arise, however, such as a student athlete/musician committing suicide on the day of a game/concert, where the "team" is in too much shock to play a game that night, and so forth). That said, supporting teachers in providing flexibility can be helpful in minimizing additional stress and burden on students who are grieving.

Common grief reactions

Common adolescent grief reactions when a peer dies by suicide include the following:

- Guilt, blaming (others and self), shame, anger, rejection, and perceived stigma
- Risky coping behaviors, such as increased alcohol consumption
- A shift in perspectives on relationships and life
- A change in level of maturity
- A need to make meaning of the suicide, and to be able to talk about their experience
- Vacillating between help-seeking behaviors and isolation[6]

Understanding how developmental differences affect the grief process in students of different ages will help guide clinicians in deciding what strategies to use and to

Table 1
Tips for talking about suicide

Give Accurate Information About Suicide	By Saying…
Suicide is a complicated behavior. It is not caused by a single event. In many cases, mental health conditions, such as depression, bipolar disorder, PTSD, or psychosis, or a substance use disorder is present leading up to a suicide. Mental health conditions affect how people feel and prevent them from thinking clearly. Having a mental health problem is actually common and nothing to be ashamed of. Help is available. Talking about suicide in a calm, straightforward way does not put the idea into people's minds.	"The cause of [NAME]'s death was suicide. Suicide is not caused by a single event. In many cases, the person has a mental health or substance use disorder and then other life issues occur at the same time leading to overwhelming mental and/or physical pain, distress, and hopelessness." "There are effective treatments to help people with mental health or substance abuse problems or who are having suicidal thoughts." "Mental health problems are not something to be ashamed of. They are a type of health issue."
Address Blaming and Scapegoating	**By Saying…**
It is common to try to answer the question "why?" after a suicide death. Sometimes this turns into blaming others for the death.	"Blaming others or the person who died does not consider the fact that the person was experiencing a lot of distress and pain. Blaming is not fair and can hurt another person deeply."
Do Not Focus on the Method	**By Saying…**
Talking in detail about the method can create images that are upsetting and can increase the risk of imitative behavior by vulnerable individuals. The focus should not be on how someone killed themselves but rather on how to cope with feelings of sadness, loss, anger, and similar	"Let's talk about how [NAME]'s death has affected you and ways you can handle it." "How can you deal with your loss and grief?"
Address Anger	**By Saying…**
Accept expressions of anger at the deceased and explain that these feelings are normal.	"It is Okay to feel angry. These feelings are normal, and it doesn't mean that you didn't care about [NAME]. You can be angry at someone's behavior and still care deeply about that person."
Address Feelings of Responsibility	**By Saying…**
Help students understand that they are not responsible for the suicide of the deceased. Reassure those who feel responsible or think they could have done something to save the deceased.	"This death is not your fault. We cannot always see the signs because a suicidal person may hide them." "We cannot always predict someone else's behavior."
Promote Help-Seeking	**By Saying…**
Encourage students to seek help from a trusted adult if they or a friend are feeling depressed.	"Seeking help is a sign of strength, not weakness." "We are always here to help you through any problem, no matter what. Who are the people you would go to if you or a friend

(continued on next page)

Table 1 (continued)	
Promote Help-Seeking	**By Saying**…
	was feeling worried or depressed or had thoughts of suicide?"
	"If you are concerned about yourself or a friend, talk with a trusted adult."

From American Foundation for Suicide Prevention, Suicide Prevention Resource Center. After a suicide: a toolkit for schools. 2nd edition. Waltham (MA): Education Development Center; 2018; with permission.

know how the death might be conceptualized. Jellinek and Okoli[12] describe developmental differences important to recognize among students at different grade levels:

- Preschool: students display "magical thinking" with little understanding about the permanence of death, sometimes seeming "casual" or even excited about rituals surrounding death. They benefit from description of positive memories of the deceased and concrete pictures or mementos.
- Elementary: students of this age are developmentally self-focused, and so they may worry about how suicide may impact them or their family. Subsequently, reassurance that they are safe and their family will not substantially change can be helpful.
- Middle school: students of this age are beginning to individuate and thus are more peer-centric as they separate from parents. They may experience feelings of concern or guilt that they should have foreseen or even prevented this death. They may benefit from a discussion of the facts surrounding the death, information they may not have had, how each peer may feel something they did (or did not do) could have influenced the suicide ("I didn't say 'hi' in the hall the day before she died—I think that may have been what pushed her over the edge."); rarely, they may have had a significant fight, breakup, episode of bullying, or efforts to oust a student from their group immediately before the suicide, and thus, may require more intensive counseling.
- High school: students can recognize the finality of this person's death and that this will be the person's "identity" in this life, so they may benefit from a discussion of the meaning of the student's life and what will persist after the funeral beyond this "article" of the person's life. Given the complexity of peer relationships at this stage, it is important to consider the nature of interpersonal relationships between the deceased and his or her peers, and especially how these factors might contribute to others' vulnerabilities.

Research indicates that adolescents experience a range of negative cognitions and emotions following a peer suicide; however, these young survivors may not always have the ability to accurately articulate or identify their thoughts and feelings. For those adolescents who do present to staff, suggesting descriptive language beyond "mad, happy, or sad" and providing education about the physiologic symptoms of emotions (ie, butterflies in the stomach, sweaty palms, fatigue, poor concentration, numbness) may be helpful. Connecting with students and keeping them engaged in talking about their emotions can help further elucidate the impact of recent events on them. Asking open-ended questions, such as, "What is your biggest concern right now?" or "What would help to make you feel safer?," will help gauge the student's current specific needs.[13,14]

> **Box 1**
> **Practical coping strategies**
>
> - Use simple relaxation and distraction skills, such as taking 3 deep slow breaths; counting to 10; or picturing themselves in a favorite calm and relaxing place
> - Engage in favorite activities or hobbies, such as music, talking with a friend, reading, or going to a movie
> - Exercise
> - Think about how they have coped with difficulties in the past and remind them that they can use those same coping skills now
> - Write a list of people they can turn to for support
> - Write a list of things they are looking forward to
> - Focus on individual goals, such as returning to a shared class or spending time with mutual friends
>
> *From* American Foundation for Suicide Prevention, Suicide Prevention Resource Center. After a suicide: a toolkit for schools. 2nd edition. Waltham (MA): Education Development Center; 2018; with permission.

Practical coping strategies

Although the experience of adolescents who are grieving a peer who died by suicide is in many ways unique, counselors and mental health professionals are familiar with effective strategies. An understanding of relaxation techniques and cognitive exercises are all helpful in promoting resiliency and healing. After a Suicide: A Toolkit for Schools makes recommendations of strategies that can help adolescents cope (**Box 1**).[10]

Meeting with students in small groups or individually and having them practice these skills in vivo can help to reduce the stigma in using coping skills and can become an experience in itself that can promote positive feelings.

Students may ask difficult questions or ones that are beyond a staff's expertise. It is ok to say, "I don't know," or to reassure the student that they will help them find the answer. Students may also ask questions that need clarification. Staff needs to make sure they get back to students with a response. Rather than quickly responding, asking students to say more about a statement can provide additional information. Finally, these small groups also serve the purpose of protecting a time and place for meaningful connections with others, which can also be therapeutic.

School routine

Students (and staff) will react differently to the suicide, such that the first week requires allowances for students to endure the natural process of grief as they contend with this event and its impact on them, their friends, and the community. Having counseling staff available throughout each day for the first week is helpful because students may appear to do well initially and then struggle over time. In addition, staff similarly needs opportunities for clinical support this first week, because they often feel exhausted at various points trying to "hold it together" for students. Pertinently, the week surrounding a student suicide is likely to be erratic, and attempting to implement the "normal routine" is often difficult for students and staff; thus, it is advised to dissuade high-stakes events (testing, sporting events, and so forth) during this interval.

Stage 2: Student Reequilibration (Weeks to Months After Suicide)

Although some students may return to baseline after the first week, other students may need several additional weeks to adjust. Flexibility may be needed both for school schedules and for individual students to resume a routine similar to the time before the suicide. Additional staff check-ins and booster support sessions may be warranted. Opportunities that will allow for students to contact school counselors/mental health staff if events rekindle painful recollections or distress that interfere with classroom functioning will still be necessary in the months following the suicide.

Some students may continue to struggle and have more impairment. Typically, 2 (often overlapping) groups of students may deteriorate or have elevated risks:

1. Students who knew the student who died by suicide
2. Students experiencing distress or psychiatric symptoms now exacerbated by this difficult event.

The interventions for each group may similarly overlap, although there are differences in response to each group.

Identifying students at risk

Students who knew the deceased student may feel inadequate, guilty, or even responsible for the suicide.[15,16] Students often perceive that they "should" have noticed some behavior or made some comment that could have prevented the suicide. Continuing to offer support at the school in the months following the event offers providers an opportunity to support these students in small groups or individual meetings. Staff and clinician efforts to listen and "hear out" the student can be particularly helpful. Clinicians or staff can then bring up other variables for consideration that may have contributed to the death. Although a suicide note might ascribe blame to another student, rarely is that the only variable contributing to a suicide.

The most common psychopathologies following a peer suicide are depression, anxiety, and posttraumatic stress disorder (PTSD), as well as an increase in suicidal behavior.[5,17–19] By understanding specific presentations of adolescent depression, anxiety, and trauma-related disorders, schools can more easily identify students who may need more support. Schools can provide screening for higher-risk individuals or for those who continue to present for help. Students who experience the suicide as traumatic and demonstrate symptoms of (1) avoidance of reminders, (2) negative cognitions (eg, the world is unsafe, it is all my fault), (3) reexperiencing of the event, and (4) difficulties with increased arousal, poor concentration, or sleep disruption a month after the event are likely struggling with PTSD and should be referred for individualized treatment. Students who are more irritable or down, suddenly doing worse in academics, and exhibiting signs of being withdrawn should be identified and screened for depression. For those who screen positive, referrals to the community are warranted, and school counselors must follow up to ensure the student was actually able to connect with the outside provider.

In addition to helping schools be on alert for psychiatric signs and symptoms, an understanding of characteristics beyond *Diagnostic and Statistical Manual of Mental Disorders* diagnoses can further identify vulnerable students. One model useful for identifying at-risk students is the "Circles of Vulnerability."[20] This trauma-derived model describes the degree of emotional impact on members of a community following the occurrence of a critical incident or disaster and can assess how suicide may impact students.[21] The 3 circles that intersect with one another are the following:

1. Psychosocial proximity,
2. Geographic proximity,
3. Populations at risk.

Understanding how students may fit in to these circles and which ones have an accumulation of risks helps to identify students who need more intensive surveillance and support.

Stage 3: School Reequilibration (Months After Suicide)

Months following the suicide, students and staff may find ways to integrate the suicide event and perhaps even be able to learn from it. The child psychiatrist can help the school recognize suicide risk factors (eg, substance use, bullying) as they consider prevention strategies. Similarly, protective factors (eg, cohesion provided by extracurricular activities, partner community groups including youth organizations, sports organizations, religious organizations) can be identified and enhanced through collaboration between the school and community leaders and organizations.

The school will typically resume the regular schedule within 1 to 2 weeks of the suicide. However, events significant to the deceased, such as roles in sporting activities, extracurricular activities, or even "anniversaries" of events or birthdays, serve as ongoing reminders and may trigger student and staff emotions. When events warrant inclusion of the student who died by suicide, early recognition and positive contributions appear most helpful. As the shock of the suicide wanes, both staff and students are positioned to think about the legacy or positive lessons this student will leave, and what viable school changes might reduce subsequent suicides in this school community.

School suicide prevention programming

Staff training to recognize and respond to student comments about suicide, death, or depression can be helpful for the "school community" to better recognize early warning signs.

Trainings useful for school staff can be found by searching in the Resources and Programs section of the SPRC Web site.

Remembrance

Anniversaries are times when students may be triggered to remember prior events and have been known to see an increase in suicidal behavior in students. Providing a positive outlet 1 year after a student suicide can help create a focus for the school community and raise awareness that help for mental health issues is available. Fund-raisers that (1) donate to a suicide prevention organization, (2) create a memory quilt in honor of the deceased, (3) organize a walk/run in the person's memory with a mental health focus, or (4) distribute materials related to mental health and suicide prevention are all ways that provide effective solutions going forward. Additional anniversaries that may trigger intense feelings include birthdays, graduation, prom, or opening day for athletic or theatrical events in which the student participated. The 2-year anniversary is also notable to students, and schools can also provide similar activities.

SUICIDE CONTAGION

Although relatively rare, suicide contagion can occur following the suicide of a peer and is often on the mind of parents and administrators in the days and weeks following. Suicide contagion can account for 1% to 5% of teenage suicides[22] or 100 to 200 deaths annually. Contagion in this context can have various meanings[21]; however, for purposes of exploring a school's response, it is defined as the process of one suicide death leading to another.[23–26] Adolescents are more susceptible to the phenomenon,[5,7,17] leading caregivers and school personnel to understandably be concerned following a student suicide. Fortunately, there are now helpful

Box 2
The role of the child psychiatrist

- Provide schools administrators with available resources for suicide postvention
- Review procedures for conducting classroom or small group presentations on responses to sudden loss
- Familiarize staff with the developmental tasks associated with recovery from loss, and the dynamic nature of trauma and loss
- Screen students and provide appropriate referrals when warranted
- Colead support groups
- Assist school staff in conducting parent meetings
- Advise staff on how to respond to media representatives
- Provide clinical consultation to school counselors and the postvention team
- Provide support services or referrals
- Meet with the postvention team to review their process
- Assist the team in evaluating their efforts
- Make suggestions for improving the postvention policy and procedures
- Identify new community resources for future situations
- Present information on prevention to community members

Adapted from Kerr MM, Brent DA, McKain B, et al. Postvention standards manual: a guide for a school's response in the aftermath of a sudden death. 4th edition. Pittsburgh (PA): University of Pittsburgh, Services for Teens at Risk (STAR-Center); 2003; with permission.

guidelines that schools can follow to help reduce the risk of suicide contagion. Well-implemented postvention can reduce further loss and trauma and lead to prevention and improved mental health among a student body. In fact, one of the goals of implementing a stronger suicide postvention response in schools is to prevent further self-harm or suicidal behavior among students in addition to supporting the student body through the experience of grief and loss.[8]

The Role of the Child Psychiatrist

Each school will adapt postvention efforts in ways that best fit their culture and climate and meet the needs of their staff and students. Child psychiatrists may serve a role in these efforts in a variety of ways. Examples of the various tasks of the child psychiatrist are described in **Box 2**.

Ultimately, incorporating mental health programming "upstream" of more well-defined problems and targeting at-risk individuals can help strengthen the emotional well-being of students. There is now ample evidence for programming to support schools in this endeavor. Schools are where children and adolescents spend most of their waking hours, and providing mental health programming, particularly in the wake of suicide and loss, can only help strengthen schools and the students within them. Although a school community that has experienced a student suicide is forever changed, in the midst of the tragedy, there is also opportunity to build resilience and maximize the potential of students, staff, administrators, and the community.

SUMMARY

When suicide occurs among school-age students, the tragedy profoundly impacts the community. The school itself is in a position to address and decrease the impact of such tragic circumstances. However, the school also benefits from community support in such an event, because this type of death requires a specialized response. High-quality, evidence-based guidelines freely available to schools can be very helpful during a devastating time for other students and staff. If called upon, child psychiatrists can provide their unique skills set and understanding of child development, psychopathology, risk assessment, as well as consultation skills to support schools throughout the crisis. Using these resources provides an effective roadmap to guide their support with a bereaved school.

REFERENCES

1. Centers for Disease Control and Prevention. 10 leading causes of death by age group, United States 2014. Available at: https://www.cdc.gov/injury/images/lc-charts/leading_causes_of_death_age_group_2014_1050w760h.gif. Accessed April 23, 2018.
2. Centers for Disease Control and Prevention. Web based injury statistics query and reporting system. 2016. Available at: https://www.cdc.gov/injury/wisqars/index.html. Accessed April 10, 2018.
3. Centers for Disease Control and Prevention. Trends in the prevalence of suicide-related behavior national YRBS: 1991-2015. 2015. Available at: https://www.cdc.gov/healthyyouth/data/yrbs/pdf/trends/2015_us_suicide_trend_yrbs.pdf. Accessed April 23, 2018.
4. Andriessen K, Rahman B, Draper B, et al. Prevalence of exposure to suicide: a meta-analysis of population-based studies. J Psychiatr Res 2017;88:113–20.
5. Gould MS, Lake AM, Kleinman M, et al. Exposure to suicide in high schools: impact on serious suicidal ideation/behavior, depression, maladaptive coping strategies, and attitudes toward help-seeking. Int J Environ Res Public Health 2018;15(3) [pii:E455].
6. Andriessen K, Draper B, Dudley M, et al. Pre- and postloss features of adolescent suicide bereavement: a systematic review. Death Stud 2016;40(4):229–46.
7. Insel BJ, Gould MS. Impact of modeling on adolescent suicidal behavior. Psychiatr Clin North Am 2008;31(2):293–316.
8. Erbacher TAS, Jonathan B, Poland S. Suicide in schools. New York: Routledge; 2015.
9. Andriessen K. Can postvention be prevention? Crisis 2009;30(1):43–7.
10. American Foundation for Suicide Prevention, Suicide Prevention Resource Center. After a suicide: a toolkit for schools. 2nd edition. Waltham (MA): Education Development Center; 2018.
11. Reporting on Suicide.org. Recommendations for reporting on suicide. 2015. Available at: http://reportingonsuicide.org/wp-content/themes/ros2015/assets/images/Recommendations-eng.pdf. Accessed April 27, 2018.
12. Jellinek MS, Okoli UD. When a student dies: organizing the school's response. Child Adolesc Psychiatr Clin N Am 2012;21(1):57–67, viii.
13. Dunne EJ, Dunne-Maxim K. Why suicide loss is different for survivors. In: Wasserman D, Wasserman C, editors. Oxford textbook of suicidology and suicide prevention: a global perspective. Oxford (United Kingdom): Oxford University Press; 2009. p. 605–8.
14. Jordan JR. Is suicide bereavement different? A reassessment of the literature. Suicide Life Threat Behav 2001;31(1):91–102.
15. Bridge JA, Day N, Day R, et al. Major depressive disorder in adolescents exposed to a friend's suicide. J Am Acad Child Adolesc Psychiatry 2003;42(11):1294–300.
16. Melhem NM, Day N, Shear MK, et al. Traumatic grief among adolescents exposed to a peer's suicide. Am J Psychiatry 2004;161(8):1411–6.

17. Brent DA, Perper JA, Moritz G, et al. Psychiatric sequelae to the loss of an adolescent peer to suicide. J Am Acad Child Adolesc Psychiatry 1993;32(3):509–17.
18. Brent DA, Perper J, Moritz G, et al. Adolescent witnesses to a peer suicide. J Am Acad Child Adolesc Psychiatry 1993;32(6):1184–8.
19. Ho TP, Leung PW, Hung SF, et al. The mental health of the peers of suicide completers and attempters. J Child Psychol Psychiatry 2000;41(3):301–8.
20. Lahad M, Cohen A. The community stress prevention center: 25 years of community stress prevention and intervention. Kiryat Shmona (Israel): The Community Stress Prevention Center; 2006.
21. Zenere F. Suicide clusters and contagion. Prinicipal Leadership 2009;10(2):12–6.
22. Lake AM, Gould MS. Suicide clusters and suicide contagion. In: Koslow S, Nemeroff C, Ruiz P, editors. A concise guide to understanding suicide: epidemiology, pathophysiology and prevention. Cambridge (United Kingdom): Cambridge University Press; 2013. p. 52–61.
23. Brent DA, Moritz G, Bridge J, et al. Long-term impact of exposure to suicide: a three-year controlled follow-up. J Am Acad Child Adolesc Psychiatry 1996; 35(5):646–53.
24. Brent DA, Perper J, Moritz G, et al. Psychiatric effects of exposure to suicide among the friends and acquaintances of adolescent suicide victims. J Am Acad Child Adolesc Psychiatry 1992;31(4):629–39.
25. Davidson LE, Rosenberg ML, Mercy JA, et al. An epidemiologic study of risk factors in two teenage suicide clusters. JAMA 1989;262(19):2687–92.
26. Cheng Q, Li H, Silenzio V, et al. Suicide contagion: a systematic review of definitions and research utility. PLoS One 2014;9(9):e108724.

Clinician Response to a Child Who Completes Suicide

Cheryl S. Al-Mateen, MD[a,b,]*, Kathryn Jones, MD, PhD[a,b], Julie Linker, PhD[a,b], Dorothy O'Keefe, MD[a,b], Valentina Cimolai, MD[a,b]

KEYWORDS

- Child • Adolescent • Suicide • Impact on clinician • Postvention • Postsuicide
- Reactions to suicide

KEY POINTS

- Suicide is the most likely cause of death for children and adolescents treated by psychiatrists. More than half of psychiatrists experience the suicide of a patient at some point in their careers.
- Psychiatrists and other clinicians often experience strong reactions to patient suicide, including shock, guilt, isolation, insomnia, and self-doubt.
- Trainees are more likely to experience the suicide of a patient and are more affected by the experience.
- Clinicians need specific training on suicide postvention, including legal, administrative, emotional, and professional ramifications.

INTRODUCTION

"There are two types of clinicians; those who have had a patient commit suicide and those who will." –Robert Simon, MD[1]

"Suicide is the major cause of mortality in the realm of diseases with which psychiatrists and other mental health clinicians work.[2]" The possibility that a child and adolescent psychiatrist will have one of their patients complete suicide is real. As many as 68% of consultant psychiatrists have lost a patient to suicide[3,4] and 22% of a group of psychologists acknowledged having a patient that completed suicide.[5] Suicide may be an occupational hazard for mental health professionals.[6]

Disclosure: The authors do not have any direct financial relationships that are related to the subject matter discussed in this article.
[a] Department of Psychiatry, Division of Child and Adolescent Psychiatry, Virginia Treatment Center for Children, Virginia Commonwealth University School of Medicine, PO Box 980489, Richmond, VA 23298, USA; [b] Department of Psychiatry, Division of Child and Adolescent Psychiatry, Virginia Treatment Center for Children, Virginia Commonwealth University School of Medicine, 1308 Sherwood Avenue, Richmond, VA 23220, USA
* Corresponding author. Virginia Treatment Center for Children, 1308 Sherwood Avenue, Richmond, VA 23220.
E-mail address: cheryl.al-mateen@vcuhealth.org

Child Adolesc Psychiatric Clin N Am 27 (2018) 621–635
https://doi.org/10.1016/j.chc.2018.05.006
1056-4993/18/© 2018 Elsevier Inc. All rights reserved.

childpsych.theclinics.com

The authors attempted to review the literature on the response of clinicians to the suicide of children and adolescents and found it lacking. Therefore, this article reviews the topic of suicide in children and adolescents, and discusses the literature on impact of suicide on mental health clinicians. From our investigation of extant literature, it is useful to consider the aftermath of a patient's suicide as a series of reactions, responsibilities, and interventions, first referred to as postvention activities.[7]

SUICIDE IN CHILDREN AND ADOLESCENTS

In our lifetime, the absolute number of deaths, as well as the age-adjusted suicide rates for all age groups except the elderly, have increased by 24%. For the youngest age group for which data exist, 10 to 14 years old, the suicide death rate has increased by 76%.[8] Thirty-five years ago, suicide was the seventh leading cause of death among children 5 to 14 years old.[9] In 2016, suicide was the second most common cause of death for those 10 to 14 years old, behind only accidental injury.[10] Because the Centers for Disease Control and Prevention National Violent Death Reporting System does not classify suicide as a cause of death for children less than 10 years of age, there are no nationwide data for younger children.[11] For decades, children were not considered to have the necessary cognitive development for suicidality, either because they lacked understanding of the lethality of their self-destructive behavior or because they did not recognize death as permanent. In a study of Canadian children,[12] 10% of first graders, 50% of third graders, and 90% of fifth graders understood the word suicide and the concept of self-initiated death. If the occurrence of suicide has increased in children older than 10 years, a similar increase in younger children seems likely, despite an absence of supportive data.

A psychological autopsy study comparing suicides in Norwegians aged 15 years and younger with matched youth killed in accidents found that only 20% of the suicides met criteria for psychiatric diagnoses and that 12% had prior suicide attempts. In retrospect, stressors were evident but at the time were not thought relevant.[13,14] A review of 15 psychological autopsy or retrospective case studies of children less than 14 years of age who died by suicide identified several unique characteristics[15] (**Box 1**).

Box 1
Literature review of 15 retrospective case studies of children less than 14 years of age who died by suicide: unique characteristics

- Gender asymmetry (male>female) in suicide is *less* marked in children than in adolescents
- Suicide is more prevalent in indigenous populations, especially in children
- Preexisting mental health diagnosis is less common in children than in older teens, as is substance use disorder, which is a significant risk factor for suicide in older adolescents
- Prior suicidal behavior in roughly 20% to 30% of completed child suicides
- Preoccupation with death (thinking, dreaming, drawing) in nearly 50%
- Family mental illness, especially past parental suicidal behavior
- Poor communication with parents; history of physical or sexual abuse
- Outside the home, academic problems and bullying contribute to increased risk
- Fewer than 20% of children who died by suicide had outpatient mental health treatment or school services in the year before their death.

Data from Soole R, Kõlves K, De Leo D. Suicide in children: a systematic review. Arch Suicide Res 2015;19(3):285–304.

The final characteristic, that less than 20% of children who die by suicide had outpatient mental health treatment or school services, is troubling. This finding suggests that children who died by suicide are among the most underserved populations with regard to mental health.

A 2008 review of studies of completed suicides of children aged 14 years and younger found that hanging is the most common method used.[16] Between 20% and 25% of those who completed suicide had previous contact with child welfare institutions. Similarly, a study of children and adolescents in the Manitoba child welfare system between 1997 and 2006 found that those in care had 4 times the risk of suicide compared with a cohort not in care, despite a decrease in suicide attempts and hospitalizations.[17]

A review of suicide deaths using National Violent Death Reporting System data from 2003 to 2012 among children aged 5 to 14 years compared by age group and race in 17 US states, widespread in location, size, and urban/rural population distributions, showed that children were more likely to be male, black, and to die by hanging or strangulation than were adolescents (12–14 years). More than one-third of the elementary school–aged children who died by suicide were black. Current mental health problems were identified in 30%, most commonly attention-deficit/hyperactivity disorder in children, whereas depression/dysthymia was more common among adolescents.[18] In most cases, interpersonal conflict precipitated the suicide; for children, this tended to be intrafamilial, such as parental loss, suicidal behavior in parents, or parental abuse.[19]

CLINICIAN RESPONSES TO SUICIDE

Fifty years ago, the discussion of suicide was taboo, even among mental health professionals.[7] In the mid-1980s, a study with extensive interviews of individuals who had lost adult family members to suicide concluded that suicide survivors had a need to talk about their loss but often lacked opportunity to do so. The investigators noted that survivors commonly experienced self-blame and guilt but also blamed others, including parents and partners of the deceased, as well as physicians and psychiatrists. They found potential for positive integration of the experience: "[the] realization of one's own limits allows for cessation of self-blame and enables the bereaved to realistically assess his or her responsibility."[20(pp205)]

In a study of parents whose children completed suicide, recurrent themes for survivors were a "wall of silence," "the absence of caring interest," and "unhelpful advice."[21(pp603)] The investigators suggested that mental health practitioners should offer guidance to survivors on how to educate their social networks to provide needed support. Such guidance would also apply to clinician survivors.

Much of the role of mental health clinicians is to ensure the safety of their patients, regardless of the level of care. However, clinicians remain unable to successfully and reproducibly predict which of their patients will not only attempt but complete suicide.[22,23] For child patients, assessment of suicide risk is even more challenging. For many years, much of the psychiatric literature held that children were incapable of experiencing depression, much less the degree of hopelessness and despair that are associated with a suicidal patient. When clinicians reexamine their conceptualization of children's emotional capacities, they find that they grossly underestimate their child patients; these patients prove themselves equally proficient at suicide as their most practiced adult counterparts.[24–26]

STAGES OF CLINICIAN ADJUSTMENT

The loss of a child or adolescent patient to suicide is devastating. Clinicians move through a landscape of emotions after a patient completes suicide. When clinicians believe they have prepared as best they can for their patients whom they know to be at high risk of completion, these feelings can be even more intense. With adolescent patients, they can sometimes with fair accuracy extrapolate lessons learned from the adult population. In contrast, the clues left by a child to point toward an understanding of their level of risk can be far subtler.[25–27] In training, clinicians were not taught what to do if a child or adolescent patient completes suicide.[28,29]

Although a great deal of the literature that was found was related to psychiatry and psychology,[5,6,30] all mental health professionals working with patients who commit suicide seems to have a similar range of reactions.[31,32] However, women were more likely to endorse feeling shame, guilt, and doubt of their professional knowledge and skills. They were also more likely to seek support from peers' supervision than male psychiatrists and psychologists.[33]

Suicide is a trauma to almost all who know the decedent.[34] In their model of determining the impact of suicide on those who have lost someone to suicide, Cerel and colleagues[35] opined that a practitioner could be in any of the following categories of survivors: exposed, affected, suicide-bereaved short term, and suicide-bereaved long term. These terms describe the range of impacts of the suicide from individuals who were acquainted with but did not know the decedent well (exposed) to those who were closely connected with the decedent and whose lives are intimately affected by the decedent's death over time (suicide bereaved). Those in the suicide-bereaved short-term category may benefit from crisis intervention or support services. Those in the long-term category may require longer support for complex grief.

A study of Thai psychiatrists found cultural differences in clinician response to patient suicide based not only on individual and regional religious beliefs but also on regional perceptions of the suicide and its causality.[4] Compared with studies of US, Scot, Australian, and German psychiatrists, the Thai psychiatrists endorsed less anger, and none considered changing professions or stopped seeing suicidal patients. These psychiatrists had fewer fears of publicity and lawsuits, and 55% attended patient funerals, which is higher than reported in the other studies.[3,30,36,37] An individual's personal and professional life experiences also affect their reactions to a patient's completed suicide.[38–40]

When a patient is lost to suicide, clinicians often believe they have unfinished business, particularly when the patient is a child or adolescent. The conversation is left unfinished; questions go unanswered except in the imagination. It is as if the clinicians' only tool (themselves, their countertransference) has failed to work.[28,34] The reflection was flawed; they did not get the message. There is the temptation for clinicians to doubt that they ever read any patient correctly, that they are not listening hard enough or in the right way. There is a small but significant literature[28,29,34] showing that patient suicide can make psychiatrists at any stage of training, but particularly early in the process, change their practice. This tendency may result in refusing to treat and to work with high-risk patients at all, and proves to be a dilemma in working with child or adolescent patients, whose levels of risk can be so difficult to determine and whose symptoms can be so challenging to interpret.

Cotton and colleagues[31] described stages of clinician adjustment after interviewing clinical staff from an inpatient unit where 4 patients completed suicide. They and others[39,41–43] note that this trauma should be treated as such. The initial stage is a crisis period, requiring support for the staff members that worked with the patient, as well as other patients who may have been on the unit[31] with the person. The primary emotions during these first few days are shock, denial, disorientation, helplessness, and confusion. The next stage spans 1 to 2 months and involves intense feelings such as depression, anxiety, rage, and guilt. It is most appropriate to hold the suicide review conference at this time, because denial and shock have subsided. In the final stage of adjustment, either new growth has occurred around the emotional scars from the trauma, resulting in healthy recovery, or prolonged disability can be recognized as a reaction to the suicide. Some of the most severe reactions are seen in those staff without professional training in mental health, those with less experience working with prolonged psychiatric disability, or those who are earlier in their careers[31] (**Box 2, Table 1**).

A study of several multidisciplinary community mental health teams and administrators working in an inner-city area of London, United Kingdom found that 86% reported experiencing at least 1 patient suicide, with an average of 4.2 suicides. Most noted that the suicide affected both their professional and personal lives, with 45% reporting effects lasting more than a month. They had increased anxiety and irritability at work, were more distant from patients, had a desire to change jobs, and avoided patients with substance abuse issues. Some noted improvement in their clinical documentation and greater likelihood of seeking support from colleagues, including via peer supervision. Only 7% took time off after the patient's death.[44]

Hendin and colleagues[45] surveyed psychologists, psychiatrists, and social workers regarding their reactions to patient suicide. Of these clinicians, one-third experienced severe distress, with high levels of depression, guilt, grief, inadequacy, and anxiety. The level of anger was also remarkably high for most therapists in the study. Female therapists, trainees, and those with less than 15 years in practice were more likely to experience severe distress. Four factors were identified that resulted in severe distress for the providers:

1. Failing to forcibly hospitalize a patient who then completed suicide
2. Having made a treatment decision that the clinician thought contributed to the suicide (such as allowing a patient to go out on a pass or giving in to parental pressure to discharge an adult patient from a group home despite an active plan)
3. Feeling blamed by the hospital administration for the suicide
4. Fear of a lawsuit.

The first 3 factors are similar to those causing distress in physicians following a medical error.[46] Although a suicide is not a medical error, the comparable experience of guilt and distress in the clinician caused by the patient's death is seen in other areas of medicine, such as obstetrics, neonatology, and oncology.[47–49] There is a connection between health care professionals working in a distressed state, reduced functionality and potential risks to patients and the work environment.[37]

Clinician reactions can be categorized as traumatic loss/grief, interpersonal relationships, and professional identity concerns.[34] The loss is not only of the patient but of the sense of safety in the treatment framework. Supervisors, current therapists,

---

Box 2
Key postvention tasks to support the clinician after a patient completes suicide

Accept that not all suicides can be prevented

Encourage staff to support each other

Normalize the experiences that the clinician is having

Formal meetings should acknowledge the stress of the event for the team/provider

Psychological autopsy should be held after the initial shock phase

Data from Refs.[2,31,44,81]

Table 1
Stages of clinician adjustment, interventions, and tasks

Period	Intervention	Time Frame	Signs and Symptoms	Tasks
Initial trauma/ personal crisis/shock	Crisis intervention for all staff, patients, families	Immediate (first few days)	• Confusion • Disorientation • Depersonalization • Disbelief • Denial • Distractibility • Fear of blame • Fear of other suicides • Helplessness • Minimal coping • Shock • Strong but undifferentiated emotional states	• Initial staff meeting to inform others and patients • Inform and support relatives of deceased patient • Protect patients on the unit; stop admissions • Contact medical examiner, police, media, hospital administrators • Attend funeral?
Turmoil	Support the team	Weeks to 2 mo	• "A flood of rage, guilt, anxiety, and depression...the most difficult and dangerous period" (Cotton et al,[31] p. 57) • Severe self-doubt • Shame, guilt • Grief, sadness, poor concentration • Sleep and appetite disturbance • Unproductive overwork • Increased absenteeism and use of sick leave • Increased alcohol intake or other self-destructive coping strategies • Overcompensation (too restrictive or too lenient) with suicidal patients • Distancing from patients/clients • Behavioral changes for clinical situations	• Suicide review conference/ psychological autopsy should be held to fully understand issues related to the suicide and focus on the staff's emotional pain and efforts • Special staff meetings and trainings
New growth/ renewed commitment	—	Several months after the suicide review conference	"Overwhelmingly intense feelings and the bitterness have passed." Cotton et al,[31] p. 58. Staff are able to pose "broad questions	—

(continued on next page)

Table 1 (continued)				
Period	Intervention	Time Frame	Signs and Symptoms	Tasks
			regarding policy, treatment and training." Cotton et al,[31] p. 58 Prolonged disability may be seen in some staff, resulting in career or job change	

Data from Refs.[31,44,56]

and previous therapists are often significant supports. Colleagues provide a sense of both support and shame; private practitioners may feel more isolated but also more latitude in how they share their experiences with others than those working in settings with more formal review processes. Risk management concerns have been described,[34] with clinicians describing internal emotional conflict when told by malpractice carriers not to discuss the case with anyone, even the patient's family or colleagues. Some practitioners took time away from work to assess and manage countertransference, and others did not. Some began to refuse suicidal referrals, whereas others hospitalized patients more quickly from anxiety related to the suicide and thought that this negatively affected their therapeutic alliance.

A survey of consultant psychiatrists in Scotland who were clinician suicide survivors found that 15% had considered early retirement, whereas 42% changed their management of suicidal patients after the event. They became more structured and cautious in their treatment planning.[3]

Stigma surrounding suicide also contributes to the clinician's level of distress.[50,51] Some may not recognize the traumatic nature of the patient's suicide to the treating clinician and doubt the legitimacy of the clinician's reaction, leading clinicians to think that they must grieve in isolation and not seek support. This outcome can delay processing the grief, which negatively affects the clinician's integration of this loss. Such stigma is associated with ongoing difficulties for suicide survivors.[21] Trauma symptoms of anxiety, general distress, numbness, and sadness related to the patient's suicide are likely to disrupt the clinician's functioning, if only temporarily, although work with other suicidal patients may trigger a recurrence.[50]

A study of German senior and trainee therapists surveyed reactions immediately, 2 weeks after, and 6 months after their patients completed suicide. This group found that ~30% of therapists experienced extreme distress, and that the immediate global distress explained much of the variance of total distress.[37] Their findings aligned with others[45,52,53] that found that trainees have more severe reactions to a patient's completed suicide. Providers who felt offended, guilty, and intensely sad, or those who remained severely distressed over time, were more likely to be extremely cautious, to make changes to their practice, and to be unable to continue to work. The strongest correlation was for feeling offended, suggesting that providers with the greatest narcissistic injury from their patient's suicide were most impaired by that suicide in terms of future practices.

TRAINEES AND PATIENT SUICIDE

Most psychiatry residents experience a patient suicide, either of someone they cared for directly, or perhaps indirectly.[29] Trainees can be expected to have the typical reactions that any clinician would have in the wake of a patient suicide: shock, anxiety, self-blame or guilt, insomnia, loss of confidence, isolation, and preoccupation with the suicide. The impact of patient suicide has consistently been shown to be more significant for trainees[54] for a variety of reasons. Trainees who are less socialized into their profession may be particularly vulnerable to negative impacts of the experience.[54] Furthermore, suicides are more likely to occur during earlier stages of training,[54] because standard psychiatry training has the least experienced residents paired with the most ill patients during rotations in emergency and inpatient services.[55] During training, when feelings of competence may be less crystallized, the sense of having possibly failed or made mistakes may be more unsettling.[56] Trainee cognitions of having greater optimism for their work, overestimating the influence they have over patients, and having less developed healthy boundaries may also increase their vulnerability.[28] For trainees and more experienced clinicians, an impact on professional functioning may result from patient suicide, with more cautious clinical decision making, avoidance of high-risk patients, or even contemplation of career changes.[57,58] There are few single events with the power to prompt such professional crises in developing clinicians. Given that junior clinicians are likely to turn to supervisors for support, it is critical that supervisors understand the impact of patient suicide and evolution of clinician reactions in order to assist the trainees in adjusting to and learning from the experience.[59]

Psychology interns, at the same stage of training as psychiatry residents, have lower rates of exposure to patients dying by suicide than psychiatry residents, likely because of curricular differences.[60] However, they experience similar patterns of distress as psychiatry trainees, comparable with patient ratings of bereavement and higher than professional psychologists.

Young age has been cited as a factor in making patient suicide particularly distressing.[58] This may relate to several factors beyond the general societal difficulty in accepting the death of a young person. Adolescent deaths by suicide are often impulsive, thus unexpected. When a trainee has an adolescent die, the age gap between the trainee and patient may be small. Speaking with a patient's family after a suicide is emotionally difficult and may have potential legal complications. However, clinicians working with children or adolescents who have died by suicide are likely to know the children's families, and may have worked with them closely, which may further increase the complexities of communication after suicide.

A national survey showed that although 91% of residency training programs provided formal training in suicide care, only 25% covered postvention,[61] and 72% of chief residents surveyed thought this topic required more attention. Psychology training programs have lower rates of structured training for working with suicidal patients but are more likely to have specific administrative, supportive, and educational postvention procedures in place.[62] The informal support of fellow colleagues, friends, and family,[57] as well as supervisors and attendings, are important in the aftermath of a patient suicide.[58] Faculty must be aware of typical reactions of trainees following a suicide and also prepared to offer both procedural and emotional support. The type of support and educational intervention changes as the trainee proceeds through various stages of grieving and adjusting postsuicide.[63] In addition to postvention, programs are beginning to successfully integrate such training into planned curricula to address the needs of emerging professionals as they work with high-risk patients[64] (**Box 3**).

> **Box 3**
> **Recommendations for training programs**
>
> Include postvention responses as part of training on suicide care early in the curriculum
> - Emphasize universality of loss of patients by suicide
> - Review postvention procedures
> - Use the interactive and evidence-based postvention teaching strategies that are becoming available
>
> Develop postvention procedures and make available to trainees and faculty. Consider including:
> - Need to seek immediate supervisory support
> - Guidelines for communication with patient's family and attendance at funeral
> - Referrals for outside supports
>
> Require training for program faculty to address education, administrative, and personal/professional consequences of patient death for trainee, to include:
> - Stages of adjusting to patient suicide
> - Addressing stigma, guilt, and self-blame
> - Need to decrease isolation
> - Need for supervisory support during programmatic or institutional reviews
> - Provide access to resources from professional and other organizations, including first-person readings or videos about postsuicide adjustment
>
> *Data from* Refs.[28,29,54,59,61,63,64]

DEBRIEFING AND ADMINISTRATIVE RESPONSIBILITIES

Although an exhaustive review of the clinician's clinical and legal responsibilities after a patient's suicide are beyond the scope of this article, there are key points. There are likely to be multiple meetings at different times in the process. In an inpatient setting, staff meetings as well as community meetings are recommended. Community meetings require that the staff provide information and support to the other patients while maintaining safety.[31] Additional staff may be needed for coverage.

There are 5 areas for psychiatrists to address after a suicide: the family, staff, other patients, risk management, and themselves,[41] although several may be addressed simultaneously. The family must be notified as soon as possible; ideally within 24 hours, privately and in a quiet setting. Family members may have a wide range of reactions and they should be given the time they need to ask questions; this is a time to convey that all that could have been done was, indeed, done for the patient, including by mental health treatment staff and any first responders, rapid response teams, or trauma center staff. Creation of a setting in which the family may safely address the range of feelings, including sadness, anger, and pain, is essential. Grief after a suicide is typically more complex and anguishing than after other deaths, which the provider can share as anticipatory guidance. Before concluding the meeting, the provider should clarify what support the family expects at this time. Collaboration with clergy can be fruitful. In contrast, if the family was already aware of the patient's suicide, the recommendation is to call the patient's family within 24 hours to offer condolences. The clinician may provide referrals for additional services for family members. Other staff working with the patient should also be informed as soon as possible.[41,65] Such proactive communication might reduce any displaced anger from the family onto the providers.

Opinions vary widely regarding attending the patient's funeral, and, although generally encouraged,[38,41] there are some caveats. Although some families welcome, and may invite, the clinician,[38] others may fault the provider for the loss of their family member.[66] Ultimately this decision should hinge on whether the clinician's attendance is helpful for the family or not,[66] because their needs are primary.

LEGAL ISSUES

After experiencing the grief of losing a patient, psychiatrists may fear having to cope with a postsuicide lawsuit, adding another layer of emotional distress. Limited data exist regarding the legal ramifications of this traumatic event.[67] There is no official estimate of the number of lawsuits filed against child and adolescent psychiatrists in the aftermath of children completing suicide and only limited anecdotal evidence of schools or school counselors who were sued.[68,69]

Mental health professionals are not considered negligent for merely failing to predict suicide, because the inability to predict suicide has been established.[23] However, it is imperative for them to demonstrate that they followed the standard of care, traditionally defined as that degree of skill and learning that is ordinarily possessed and exercised by members of that profession in good standing. Regarding suicide, the standard of care involves assessment of the relative degree of suicide risk and development of a treatment and safety plan consistent with that risk.[70] Clinicians must understand basic principles behind a malpractice claim and be prepared with proper and systematic documentation,[67,71] with clear evaluation of suicide risk and documentation of risk factors, including prior attempts and feelings of hopelessness, as well as of protective factors. Such documentation is critical and can prevent cases from proceeding. In the inpatient setting, documentation justifying specific suicide precautions will be crucial if suicide is completed in the hospital. Moreover, before discharge, because about 25% of patients do not admit suicidal ideation to their health care provider, documentation of what the patient reports,[72] as well as objective signs of improvement (ie, improved appetite and/or sleeping, group therapy participation, and brighter affect), are critical.[73]

Hospital and agency providers must apprise themselves of their institution's standard operating procedures in this situation. Immediate supervisors must be informed, as well as risk management and malpractice insurance carriers, as soon as possible. The patient's medical record must be updated, describing the facts surrounding the suicide as they occurred and dating these entries to the medical record accurately, without drawing conclusions, apologizing, or justifying any treatment decisions, with clarification that these notes were entered after the suicide. It is wise to seek legal counsel, who should be considered and involved at all stages.[65,67]

SUMMARY

There is little statistical information about suicide in children because of long-held perceptions that children less than 10 years of age are not able to deliberately plan a suicide. No current literature exists describing the reactions of child and adolescent mental health providers to the completed suicide of their patients. Those clinicians

---

Box 4
Impact of patient suicide on mental health providers working with children and adolescents: take-home points

This is an occupational risk for all mental health providers

It is a traumatic event for all providers that requires increased care for those in training

Training for mental health providers should include a review of the topic

Suicide case conferences should consider the timing of the event and provide as much support as possible to the clinicians

Clinicians should not go through this alone; colleagues are an extremely important resource, as are families and friends

---

Box 5
Resources for clinicians who have had a patient commit suicide

Grief after Suicide[51]

American Association of Suicidology; Clinician Survivors http://www.suicidology.org/suicide-survivors/clinician-survivors

The September 2005 issue of *Women and Therapy* contains several first-person clinical survivor accounts to help other survivor clinicians[74–80]

---

exhibiting the greatest distress after a patient's completed suicide may have more guilt or anger, which may lead to greater difficulty resolving their grief regarding the patient. These clinicians need more support in coping with this trauma to minimize progression to depression or burnout, resulting in the loss of highly skilled mental health providers (**Boxes 4** and **5**).

ACKNOWLEDGMENTS

The authors would like to acknowledge Daina Ngugi, MD, for her assistance with this article.

REFERENCES

1. Simon RI. Psychiatrists awake! suicide risk assessments are all about a good night's sleep. Psychiatr Ann 1998;28(9):479–85.
2. Plakun EM, Tillman JG. Responding to clinicians after loss of a patient to suicide. Dir Psychiatry 2005;25:10. Available at: http://www.austenriggs.org/sites/default/files/resources/EMP%20%26%20JT_Responding%20to%20Clinicians%20After%20Loss%20of%20a%20Patient%20to%20Suicide.pdf. Accessed March 15, 2018.
3. Alexander DA, Klein S, Gray NM, et al. Suicide by patients: questionnaire study of its effect on consultant psychiatrists. BMJ 2000;320(7249):1571–4.
4. Thomyangkoon P, Leenaars A. Impact of death by suicide of patients on Thai psychiatrists. Suicide Life Threat Behav 2008;38(6):728–40.
5. Chemtob CM, Hamada RS, Bauer G, et al. Patient suicide: frequency and impact on psychologists. Prof Psychol Res Pract 1988;19(4):416.
6. Chemtob CM, Bauer GB, Hamada RS, et al. Patient suicide: occupational hazard for psychologists and psychiatrists. Prof Psychol Res Pract 1989;20(5):294.
7. Shneidman ES. Prologue: fifty-eight years. In: Shneidman ES, editor. On the nature of suicide. San Francisco (CA): Jossey-Bass; 1969. p. 1–30.
8. Curtin S, Warner M, Hedegaard H. Suicide rates for females and males by race and ethnicity: United States, 1999 and 2014. NCHS Health E-Stat. Atlanta (GA): National Center for Health Statistics; 2016. Available at: https://www.cdc.gov/nchs/data/hestat/suicide/rates_1999_2014.pdf. Accessed March 18, 2018.
9. Pfeffer CR. The suicidal child. New York: The Guilford Press; 1986. p. 24.
10. Centers for Disease Control and Prevention, National Center for Injury Prevention and Control. Web-based Injury Statistics Query and Reporting System (WISQARS). 2005. Available at: www.cdc.gov/injury/wisqars. Accessed March 26, 2018.
11. Centers for Disease Control and Prevention. National Violent Death Reporting System (NVDRS) searches.pdf. National Violent Death Reporting System. Available at: https://wisqars.cdc.gov:8443/nvdrs/nvdrsDisplay.jsp. Accessed March 26, 2018.

12. Normand CL, Mishara BL. The development of the concept of suicide in children. Omega: Journal of Death and Dying 1992;25:183–203.
13. Freuchen A, Kjelsberg E, Lundervold AJ, et al. Differences between children and adolescents who commit suicide and their peers: a psychological autopsy of suicide victims compared to accident victims and a community sample. Child Adolesc Psychiatry Ment Health 2012;6(1):1.
14. Freuchen A, Kjelsberg E, Lundervold AJ, et al. Correction: differences between children and adolescents who commit suicide and their peers: a psychological autopsy of suicide victims compared to accident victims and a community sample. Child Adolesc Psychiatry Ment Health 2013;7(1):18.
15. Soole R, Kolves K, DeLeo D. Suicide in children: a systematic review. Arch Suicide Res 2015;19:285–304.
16. Dervic K, Brent D, Oquendo M. Completed suicide in childhood. Psychiatr Clin North Am 2008;31:271–91.
17. Katz L, Au W, Singal D, et al. Suicide and suicide attempts in children and adolescents in the child welfare system. Can Med Assoc J 2011;183:1977–81.
18. Sheftall A, Asti L, Horowitz L, et al. Suicide in elementary school-aged children and early adolescents. Pediatrics 2016;138:e20160436.
19. Pfeffer CR. Childhood suicidal behavior: a developmental perspective. Psychiatr Clin North Am 1997;20:551–62.
20. Dunn RG, Morrish-Vidners D. The psychological and social experience of suicide survivors. Omega (Westport) 1988;18(3):175–215.
21. Feigelman W, Gorman BS, Jordan JR. Stigmatization and suicide bereavement. Death Stud 2009;33(7):591–608.
22. Pokorny AD. Prediction of suicide in psychiatric patients. Arch Gen Psychiatry 1983;40:249–57.
23. Pokorny AD. Suicide prediction revisited. Suicide Life Threat Behav 1993;23: 1–10.
24. Myllykangas M, Parhi K. The unjustified emotions: child suicide in Finnish psychiatry from the 1930s until the 1970s. J Hist Child Youth 2016;9(3):489–508.
25. Tishler C, Reiss N, Rhodes A, et al. Suicidal behavior in children younger than twelve: a diagnostic challenge for emergency department personnel. Acad Emerg Med 2007;14:810–8.
26. Pompili M, Mancinelli I, Girardi P, et al. Childhood suicide: a major issue in pediatric health care. Issues Compr Pediatr Nurs 2005;28:63–8.
27. Parrish M, Tunkle J. Clinical challenges following an adolescent's death by suicide: bereavement issues faced by family, friends, schools, and clinicians. Clin Soc Work J 2005;33(1):81–102.
28. Ellis T, Patel A. Client suicide: what now? Cogn Behav Pract 2012;19:277–87.
29. Jadhav S, Chandra P, Saranga V. Unexpected death or suicide by a child or adolescent: improving responses and preparedness of child and adolescent psychiatry trainees. Innov Clin Neurosci 2011;8(11):15–9.
30. Chemtob CM, Hamada RS, Bauer G, et al. Patients' suicides: frequency and impact on psychiatrists. Am J Psychiatry 1988;145(2):224.
31. Cotton PG, Drake RE, Whitaker A, et al. Dealing with suicide on a psychiatric inpatient unit. Hosp Community Psychiatry 1983;34(1):55–8.
32. Valente SM. Psychotherapist reactions to the suicide of a patient. Am J Orthopsychiatry 1994;64(4):614–21.
33. Grad OT, Zavasnik A, Groleger U. Suicide of a patient: gender differences in bereavement reactions of therapists. Suicide Life Threat Behav 1997;27(4): 379–86.

34. Tillman JG. When a patient commits suicide: an empirical study of psychoanalytic clinicians. Int J Psychoanal 2006;87(1):159–77.
35. Cerel J, McIntosh JL, Neimeyer RA, et al. The continuum of "survivorship": definitional issues in the aftermath of suicide. Suicide Life Threat Behav 2014;44(6): 591–600.
36. Trimble L, Jackson K, Harvey D. Client suicidal behaviour: impact, interventions, and implications for psychologists. Aust Psychol 2000;35(3):227–32.
37. Wurst FM, Kunz I, Skipper G, et al. The therapist's reaction to a patient's suicide: results of a survey and implications for health care professionals' well-being. Crisis 2011;32(2):99–105.
38. Markowitz JC. Attending the funeral of a patient who commits suicide. Am J Psychiatry 1990;147(1):122–3.
39. Horn PJ. Therapists' psychological adaptation to client suicide. Psychother Theor Res Pract Train 1994;31(1):190–5.
40. Valente SM, Saunders JM. Nurses' grief reactions to a patient's suicide. Perspect Psychiatr Care 2009;38(1):5–14.
41. Kaye NS, Soreff SM. The psychiatrist's role, responses, and responsibilities when a patient commits suicide. Am J Psychiatry 1991;148(6):739.
42. Menninger WW. Patient suicide and its impact on the psychotherapist. Bull Menninger Clin 1991;55(2):216–27.
43. Little JD. Staff response to inpatient and outpatient suicide: what happened and what do we do? Aust N Z J Psychiatry 1992;26(2):162–7.
44. Linke S, Wojciak J, Day S. The impact of suicide on community mental health teams: findings and recommendations. Psychiatr Bull 2002;26(02):50–2.
45. Hendin H, Haas AP, Maltsberger JT, et al. Factors contributing to therapists' distress after the suicide of a patient. Am J Psychiatry 2004;161(8):1442–6.
46. Schwappach DLB, Boluarte TA. The emotional impact of medical error involvement on physicians: a call for leadership and organisational accountability. Swiss Medical Weekly 2008;138(1–2):9–15.
47. Meier DE. The inner life of physicians and care of the seriously Ill. JAMA 2001; 286(23):3007.
48. Shanafelt T, Adjei A, Meyskens FL. When your favorite patient relapses: physician grief and well-being in the practice of oncology. J Clin Oncol 2003;21(13):2616–9.
49. Gold KJ, Kuznia AL, Hayward RA. How physicians cope with stillbirth or neonatal death: a national survey of obstetricians. Obstet Gynecol 2008;112(1):29–34.
50. Gutin N, McGann V, Jordan JR. The impact of suicide on professional caregivers. In: Jordan JR, McIntosh JL, editors. Grief after suicide - understanding the consequences and caring for the survivors. 1st edition. New York: Routledge; 2011. p. 93–112.
51. Jordan JR, McIntosh JL, editors. Grief after suicide – understanding the consequences and caring for the survivors. 1st edition. New York: Routledge; 2011.
52. Foster VA, McAdams CR. The impact of client suicide in counselor training: implications for counselor education and supervision. Counselor Education and Supervision 1999;39(1):22–33.
53. Hendin H, Lipschitz A, Maltsberger JT, et al. Therapists' reactions to patients' suicides. Am J Psychiatry 2000;157(12):2022–7.
54. Ruskin R, Sakinofsky I, Bagby R, et al. Impact of patient suicide on psychiatrists and psychiatric trainees. Acad Psychiatry 2004;28(2):104–10.
55. Fang F, Kemp J, Jawandha A, et al. Encountering patient suicide: a resident's experience. Acad Psychiatry 2007;31:340–4.

56. Gitlin M. Aftermath of a tragedy - reaction of psychiatrists to patient suicides. Psychiatr Ann 2007;37(10):684–7.
57. Pilkinton P, Etkin M. Encountering suicide: the experience of psychiatric residents. Acad Psychiatry 2003;27(2):93–9.
58. Dewar I, Eagles J, Klein S, et al. Psychiatric trainees' experiences of, and reactions to, patient suicide. Psychiatr Bull 2000;24:20–3.
59. Kleepsies P. The stress of patient suicidal behavior: implications for interns and training programs in psychology. Prof Psychol Res Pract 1993;24(4):477–82.
60. Kleepsies P, Smith M, Becker B. Psychology interns as patient suicide survivors: incidence, impact, and recovery. Prof Psychol Res Pract 1990;21(4):257–63.
61. Melton B, Coverdale J. What do we teach psychiatric residents about suicide: a national survey of chief residents. Acad Psychiatry 2009;33:47–50.
62. Ellis T, Dickey T. Procedures surrounding the suicide of a trainee's patient: a national survey of psychology internships and psychiatry residency programs. Prof Psychol Res Pract 1998;29(5):493–7.
63. Brown H. Patient suicide during residency training: incidence, implications, and program response. J Psychiatry 1987;11:201–6.
64. Prabhakar D, Balon R, Anzia J, et al. Helping psychiatry residents cope with patient suicide. Acad Psychiatry 2014;38(5):593–7.
65. Jain S, Jain R. Key steps to take when a patient commits suicide. Curr Psychiatr 2014;13(2):78–9.
66. Freedenthal S. Should therapists attend the funeral of a client who dies by suicide.pdf. Speaking of Suicide. 2013. Available at: https://www.speakingofsuicide.com/2013/08/07/funeral-after-client-suicide/. Accessed March 4, 2018.
67. Feldman SR, Moritz SH, Benjamin GAH. Suicide and the law: a practical overview for mental health professionals. Women Ther 2004;28(1):95–103.
68. Balingit M. Parents of Virginia teen who committed suicide sue school counselor. Washington Post 2016. Available at: https://www.washingtonpost.com/local/education/parents-of-teen-who-committed-suicide-sue-school-counselor/2016/12/03/f417bfae-b975-11e6-a677-b608fbb3aaf6_story.html?utm_term=.6531c0f911c9. Accessed March 2, 2018.
69. Schmidt S. After months of bullying, her parents say a 12 year old New Jersey girl killed herself. They blame the school. The Washington Post 2017. Available at: https://www.washingtonpost.com/news/morning-mix/wp/2017/08/02/after-months-of-bullying-a-12-year-old-new-jersey-girl-killed-herself-her-parents-blame-the-school/?utm_term=.a90b37b76364. Accessed March 24, 2018.
70. Packman WL, O'Connor Pennuto T, Bongar B, et al. Legal issues of professional negligence in suicide cases. Behav Sci Law 2004;22(5):697–713.
71. Sher L. Suicide medical malpractice: an educational overview. Int J Adolesc Med Health 2015;27(2):203–6.
72. Simon RI. Suicide risk assessment forms: form over substance? J Am Acad Psychiatry Law 2009;37(3):4.
73. Partridge M. Strategies to avoid a malpractice suit when a patient commits suicide. Psychiatr Times 2009;26:11. Available at: http://www.psychiatrictimes.com/articles/strategies-avoid-malpractice-suit-when-patient-commits-suicide. Accessed March 19, 2018.
74. Weiner KM. Introduction: the professional is personal. Women Ther 2004;28(1):1–7.
75. James DM. Surpassing the quota: multiple suicides in a psychotherapy practice. Women Ther 2004;28(1):9–24.
76. Anderson GO. Who, what, when, where, how, and mostly why?: a therapist's grief over the suicide of a client. Women Ther 2004;28(1):25–34.

77. Spiegelman JS, Werth JL. Don't forget about me: the experiences of therapists-in-training after a client has attempted or died by suicide. Women Ther 2004;28(1): 35–57.
78. Schultz D. Suggestions for supervisors when a therapist experiences a client's suicide. Women Ther 2004;28(1):59–69.
79. Grad OT, Michel K. Therapists as client suicide survivors. Women Ther 2004; 28(1):71–81.
80. Rycroft P. Touching the heart and soul of therapy: surviving client suicide. Women Ther 2004;28(1):83–94.
81. Farrington A. Suicide and psychological debriefing. Br J Nurs 1995;4(4):209–11.

CPI Antony Rowe
Chippenham, UK
2019-02-06 16:07